# Dr Eva Orsmond's Reverse Your Diabetes

*The Revolutionary Diet Plan for Taking Control of Type 2 Diabetes*

GILL BOOKS

**Gill Books**
Hume Avenue
Park West
Dublin 12
www.gillbooks.ie

Gill Books is an imprint of M.H. Gill and Co.

978 07171 8132 2

Designed by Graham Thew
Edited by Rachel Pierce and Kristin Jensen
Proofread by Jane Rogers
Indexed by Eileen O'Neill
Photography by Monika Coghlan
Photo on p. vi courtesy of *Irish Daily Mail*
Photo on p. 112 courtesy of iStock/Getty Premium
Illustrations on pp. 8 and 9 by Derry Dillon
Styling by Claire Wilkinson
Printed by BZ Graf, Poland
This book is typeset in Freight Micro Pro Book, 10.5 on 14pt.

The paper used in this book comes from the wood pulp of managed forests. For every tree felled, at least one tree is planted, thereby renewing natural resources.

A CIP catalogue record for this book is available from the British Library.

5 4 3 2 1

ACKNOWLEDGEMENTS

Alone we can do so little; together we can do so much. This book is a prime example of great team work.

First and most importantly I want to thank Wyatt, my best friend and husband of many years, for sticking with me through thick and thin. Without you this book would not be here. We've had (have!) our challenges but you have always supported me with my work and life aspirations and goals, and I love and thank you for that.

Thank you to my wonderful teams in my clinics, who have all contributed to making this book – for the recipes we have perfected together over the years and the support and inspiration we have given each other. And most importantly thank you to the many patients we have seen over the years looking to improve their health, particularly those who agreed to share their stories in this book. A special thank you to Katri for her loyalty, hard work and her sincere and honest opinions. Finnish SISU at its best.

There are many people in the media to whom I owe a big thank you. The teams at the *Irish Daily Mail*, *Irish Examiner*, *Irish Independent*, *Irish Times*, *Limerick Leader*, *Sunday Business Post*, *Clare Byrne Live*, *Ireland AM*, Newstalk, the *Pat Kenny Show*, the *Six O'Clock Show*, *Sunday AM* (Virgin Media One, previously TV3), Ray D'Arcy in RTÉ and many more who have supported me on this long road to get the truth out there.

A special thanks to Gill Books for believing in me and publishing this book, which goes against the grain and takes us back to the basics of addressing the cause of the problem and not the symptoms.

ABOUT THE AUTHOR

**Dr Eva Orsmond, MD MPH,** is a medical doctor with a special interest in weight management and the treatment of overweight and obese adults and children. She appeared for a number of years on RTÉ's popular *Operation Transformation*, and also presented the widely watched television documentaries, *Sugar Crash* and *Medication Nation*. Her two previous books, *The Last Diet* and *The 10lb Diet*, were bestsellers.

NOTE

Any person with a condition requiring medical attention should consult their GP or a qualified medical practitioner.

# Contents

001 ............ Preface

004 ............ **Introduction**
007 ............ Where Do We Go From Here?
011 ............ Case Studies
032 ............ What is Diabetes Mellitus?
047 ............ The Role of Smoking and Alcohol
050 ............ Driving and Diabetes
053 ............ Diabetes Medication and its Side-Effects
061 ............ Very Low-Calorie Ketogenic Diet (VLCKD) Explained
068 ............ What to Expect
072 ............ The Plan
074 ............ Phase 1
078 ............ Phase 2
082 ............ Phase 3
087 ............ Maintenance

095 ............ **The Recipes**
101 ............ Breakfast
117 ............ Lunch
133 ............ Soups and Salads
149 ............ Dinner
195 ............ Carbohydrate Substitutes
205 ............ Vegetable Side Dishes
219 ............ Dessert

227 ............ Appendix
228 ............ Index

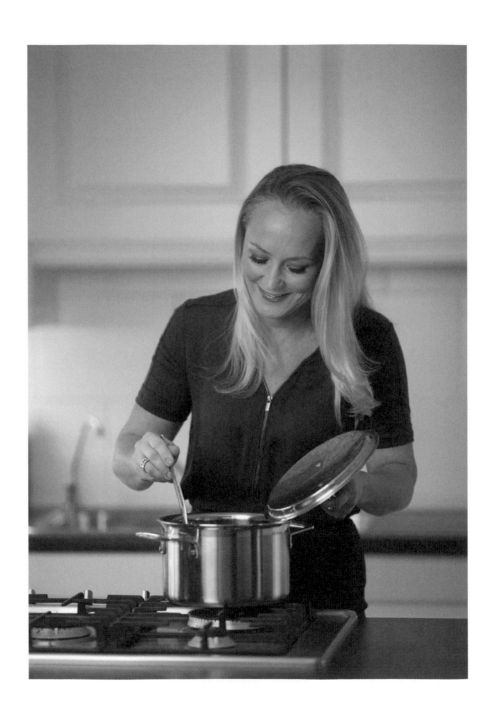

# Preface

When we are young, we are often idealistic, believing in the possibility of changing the world for the better. I was such a young idealist, and I wanted to become a doctor with the enthusiasm that drives so many aspiring students. The Hippocratic Oath was the ultimate goal I aspired to.

When I entered clinical practice, I came face-to-face with reality when the consultant I was working under said to me: 'Half of the symptoms patients complain about are not serious (life-threatening) and we will sort them out, and the other half we can't do anything about anyhow.' Slowly but surely, I was introduced to the bleak reality of modern medicine, where pharmaceutical drugs are almost the only treatment option. Over the years of my medical studies, I had been taught that as doctors we should treat the *cause* of the disease, not the symptoms, but once I entered clinical practice I saw very little of that. My expectations did not meet reality.

As I worked and gained experience and witnessed healthcare first-hand, I was struck by how many people have a blind trust in doctors. So many people treat doctors with a sort of reverence, as if they have a knowledge and an understanding far beyond the rest of us. This is not the case.

This is an important thing to understand – medicine is not a secret science. Look for information and be informed. In Ireland, people don't ask enough questions or seek second opinions. I have heard the same story again and again from my patients over the years: that their doctor failed to listen to them and, as a consequence, their diagnosis was delayed while they became even sicker (see Tom Treacy case study, p.21); or that they were just given pills and sent away. If this book makes you more determined to get informed, be informed and stay informed, I'll be very happy indeed.

From the outset, I was disappointed by this symptom-led approach to medicine in Ireland. I was looking for a more holistic view on the patient's needs. It was at a later stage in my public health studies that obesity was highlighted as a new epidemic that would cost millions to governments around the world. I decided to do my Master's degree on the problem of overweight and obesity. This turned out to be a watershed moment in my career because it was then that I realised the need for medically supervised weight management, which led to the opening of my first weight-loss clinic in 2001.

My interest in and passion for type 2 diabetes developed quite accidentally. Initially, the diet options I offered for patients were calorie-counted, based on low glycaemic index, which was a new concept at the time. I helped patients with different chronic conditions to lose weight, including diabetics (types 1 and 2). It became clear to me that weight loss was a very effective way to improve and manage health. In 2003 I went to a (pharmaceutically sponsored) diabetes conference in Finland, and that kick-started my interest in the very low-calorie ketogenic diet (VLCKD). After discussing the VLCKD and its use in type 2 diabetes with my Finnish colleagues at the conference, I became convinced that it was the best approach and started to investigate how I could introduce it into my clinics. I met with the food supplement company Eurodiet soon after my return to Ireland and heard how their products could be used to induce ketosis, while at the same time providing my patients with the vitamins and minerals needed on a daily basis to maintain good health. I ordered my first batch of food supplements and started to introduce them gradually to my weight-loss patients.

I have had great success with the Eurodiet range because they offer such a wide variety of products, so usually all of my patients can find something they enjoy from the range. I must disclose, however, that I sell them through my clinic. They are my brand of choice, but there are alternative brands available, which I have listed in the Appendix on p. 227. However, I have not tried any of these as I have built up my experience using Eurodiet and stick with what I know.

I have now been helping people to lose weight and reverse their type 2 diabetes with this diet for more than 15 years. My patients' outcomes prove that the VLCKD works, and that the benefits are far-reaching. I have included some personal patient stories in the Case Studies section (p. 11), and these true life experiences describe just how effective this approach is in tackling type 2 diabetes. That is why I'm so happy to have the opportunity to write this book and help people suffering from type 2 diabetes to take control of their illness. I'm here to tell you that it is not hopeless – you can improve your health and lifestyle by making a few dietary changes that will lead to big results!

This book aims to give you more information about the disease you dread becoming affected by, or have already been diagnosed with. Once equipped with knowledge and the message of hope, you will be in a better position to make decisions about the way you want to lead your life. I hope you read this book, from beginning to end, before embarking on any changes. You will most likely feel hugely motivated and want to start the diet immediately after reading the inspiring Case Studies section, but you must 'hold your horses' until you have acquired more knowledge, because knowledge is power.

I would also advise you to talk to your healthcare professionals, e.g. your GP, diabetic nurse specialist or consultant endocrinologist, and ask them to assist you in your journey to health and a drug-free life.

I am very negative in many sections of this book about some of my colleagues' attitudes and the way some of them practise medicine, but I am not anti doctors. I am anti bad medicine. There are many progressive, modern, open-minded doctors and consultants and nurses out there. Not only will you have a bigger chance of succeeding if you surround yourself with a network of support, you also need professional help to reduce your medications when you embark on this journey.

Preparation is the key to success. First, read this book and then, equipped with your new knowledge, look for support and help from your healthcare provider. After that you are already half-way there because good planning is half the job.

Good luck and God bless. You can do it!

# Introduction
## Diabetes in Ireland: what should change?

We are all too often led to believe that type 2 diabetes mellitus is a condition whereby the body does not make enough insulin, and that the insulin produced doesn't work as well as it should. The truth is, type 2 diabetes starts as insulin resistance and only with time and an unchanged lifestyle does it eventually lead to insulin exhaustion.

The role that excess weight and abdominal obesity play in type 2 diabetes is rarely discussed. The idea of taking personal responsibility for this excess weight and encouraging people to do something about it is a topic that is seldom, if ever, raised. Instead, people are nudged in the direction of a life where they 'manage' their condition with medication, and not just medication for their diabetes but for all the other ailments that go hand in hand with it.

While age and genetics play a role in the development of type 2 diabetes, the *real* cause is excessive visceral fat ('deep' fat that surrounds internal organs) in the abdomen, which leads to insulin resistance. I often wonder why this important information is never included in government-funded type 2 diabetes websites or literature made available to diabetics and the general public. Instead, the advice focuses on treating the symptoms of the disease, not the underlying cause. If type 2 diabetes is caused by excess visceral fat produced as a result of excess weight, surely the treatment should be changes in diet and lifestyle that result in weight loss? Or is that too simplistic? Well, I don't think it is, and neither does the International Diabetes Federation (IDF), whose *Clinical Practice Recommendations for Managing Type 2 Diabetes in Primary Care* states that weight loss and lifestyle change should be the first line of treatment: 'In many cases, type 2 diabetes can be prevented by adopting a healthy lifestyle. Much can be done to improve the quality of life, increase physical activity, and reduce morbidity and mortality in people living with diabetes' (*Clinical Practice Recommendations,* p. 3).

There is plenty of research showing that changing your diet to lose visceral fat can actually *reverse* your type 2 diabetes (e.g. the DiRECT study by Professor Roy Taylor (Taylor *et al.* in *The Lancet*, DOI: 10.1016/S0140-6736(17)33102-1, December 2017)). So why isn't everyone shouting this from the rooftops? I have come to the conclusion that there are too many people and organisations with a vested interest in the treatment method of type 2 diabetes, including doctors, public health officials, the food industry and pharmaceutical companies, who have a lot to gain economically by not making the necessary changes that would have a profound impact on every type 2 diabetic in this country.

Even as I write this, the government is being encouraged to deal with the diabetes crisis using the usual 'quick fixes'. Bariatric surgery (the surgical reduction of the size of the stomach to aid weight loss), while it has a role in the treatment of obesity, is not the solution for most people. Again, this solution to obesity is treating the symptoms and not getting to the cause! Education, support and services for those who want a real alternative are hard to come by. In this, we could learn something from Finland, where patients attend regular state-run, medically led weight management classes in groups before they are placed on the waiting list for bariatric surgery – unless they have first tried the VLCKD.

The way we deal with diabetes in Ireland today is truly horrendous. There is no national diabetes register, which means that we do not have definitive data on the number of people living with the condition. This data is essential if Ireland is to deliver good chronic disease management to type 2 diabetics. Healthcare providers are also not equipped to deliver preventive programmes for high-risk patients or to educate newly diagnosed diabetics about lifestyle changes that would reverse the condition and avoid the dreaded complications. The eighth edition of the *IDF Diabetes Atlas*, published on 14 November 2017, estimates that in Ireland there are 164,984 people (4.65% of the population) living with type 1 or type 2 diabetes, and that an unbelievable 77,983 people remain undiagnosed. It is important to note that lumping type 1 and type 2 diabetes into the same group of statistics is wrong: type 1 diabetics have no choice but to live with the disease; but type 2 diabetics do have choices and can even reverse their condition if they make the decision to deal with it head-on.

The IDF estimates that the number of deaths attributed to diabetes in Ireland in 2017 was 1,091, with the average spend on each diabetic patient being just under €6,000 pa.

The above figures are either estimates or self-reported data, which means that solid, researched data is not available for Ireland. This is difficult to believe when we are talking about a disease that is taking, on average, 10% of the healthcare budget (according to Department of Health figures).

New in the 2017 *IDF Diabetes Atlas* is a chapter on the growing burden of diabetes complications, which can be life-threatening and are associated with both increased healthcare costs and reduced quality of life. Such complications can include cardiovascular disease, nephropathy (kidney disease), retinopathy (which leads to eyesight deterioration), neuropathy (chronic general pains – microvascular disease), as well as diabetic foot disease, oral health and pregnancy-related complications. Risk of cardiovascular disease in people with diabetes increases by two to three times. Risk of lower-limb amputation is increased by 10 to 20 times. Risk of developing end-stage renal disease (ESRD) is increased by ten times. One in three people with diabetes will develop retinopathy.

So what does this mean financially? We spend €153 million each year, according to the Department of Health, fighting a lifestyle disease that is largely self-inflicted.

And then there is the personal cost to diabetics, some of whom end up losing their jobs due to complications from the disease. To think that there are 425 million people around the world (2017 figures) who are either suffering from these complications or are at a high risk of developing them is very sad. And even more frightening is that these figures are increasing rapidly every day around the globe.

The growth of this disease has reached epidemic proportions around the world, and Ireland has not escaped. There has been a doubling of the prevalence of diabetes in Ireland since 1998. Traditionally, diabetes was more common in older people, affecting more than one in ten adults aged 55+. This led to the disease being referred to as 'adult onset diabetes', but its name was changed to 'type 2 diabetes' to reflect the lower age profile of those now being diagnosed. Frighteningly, there has been a marked increase in diabetes in the 18–44 age group, and this trend continues to grow. This is a

shocking development, and it is imperative that we educate and support people of all ages so they can avoid acquiring type 2 diabetes in the first place.

So why, then, is more not being done to show those with type 2 diabetes that they do not need to take medication for the rest of their lives? From the outset there is no financial motivation. In Ireland, they are provided with free medication under the Long-Term Illness Scheme, free retinal screening and in some cases a medical card, but where is the emphasis on curing this disease through weight loss and dietary change? Where is the personal responsibility?

Under the Long-Term Illness Scheme, there is no distinction between type 1 and type 2 diabetes; it just lists diabetes mellitus. In my opinion this is incorrect as type 2 diabetes does not need to be lifelong and it is a condition which is lifestyle related. Only type 1 diabetes should be on the list.

# Where Do We Go From Here?

Once we understand the cause of this disease, we can begin to treat it in an effective way. So what should we do?

First and foremost, we need to give people the correct information and advice about type 2 diabetes. The current, misleading definition of type 2 diabetes would be the first to go. This is the definition that says 'diabetes is a chronic progressive disease – chronic because you have it for ever and progressive because it will only get worse'.

This should be replaced with a more up-to-date, science-based and educational definition that points the finger of blame directly where it belongs: the excess fat in the middle of our bodies. We need to stop calling it a chronic progressive disease. It is only 'progressive' if the person *remains* overweight or obese. We need to emphatically stress to people that this disease doesn't appear from nowhere; that lifestyle is the main contributing factor. Poor food choices make you overweight, the excess weight creates visceral fat, the visceral fat results in insulin resistance, and insulin resistance results in type 2 diabetes. That's the chain of causation.

We need to start telling people that the most effective treatment is *not* drugs but weight loss. Weight loss gets to the root cause of this disease and halts it; drugs just delay the progression of the disease – they don't stop it.

In order to move towards the correct advice, I would also make further changes to the recently updated food pyramid. While the changes made to the food pyramid under the New National Obesity Strategy were welcome, they did not go far enough: placing vegetables at the bottom and moving carbohydrates up *one* level is tokenistic at best. Dietitians are using this 'updated' food pyramid in government-funded diabetes clinics throughout the country. It recommends 4–5 servings of carbohydrates every day, despite evidence that shows that type 2 diabetics are intolerant to carbohydrates!

Dr Eva's food pyramid model goes much further: vegetables form the base, followed by protein, then starch with fruit, and treats at the top.

# The Irish Food Pyramid

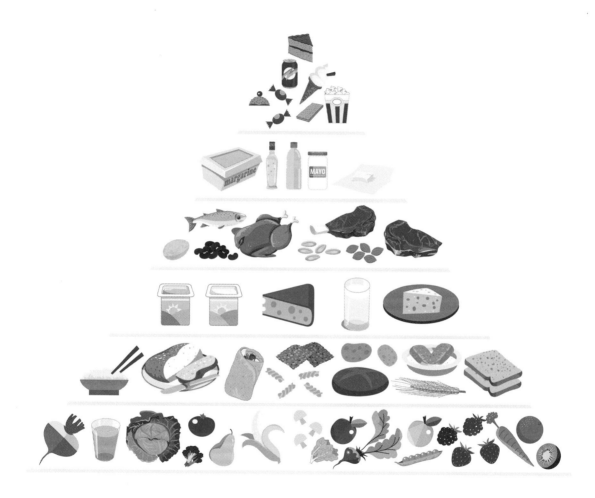

# Dr Eva's Food Pyramid

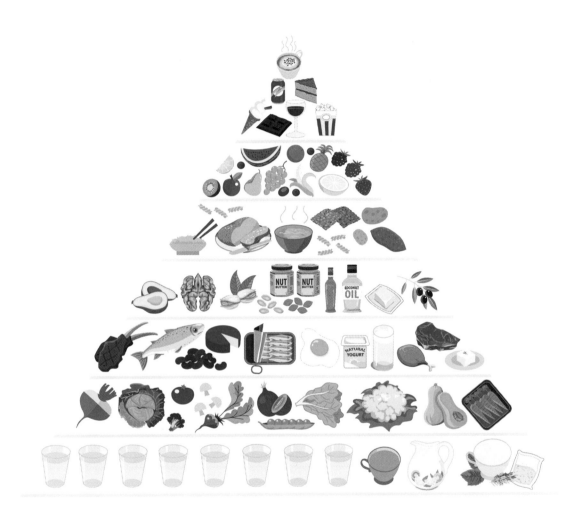

The recently updated guidelines in Ireland are already out of date. The food pyramid still promotes getting the majority of your energy from unrefined and wholegrain starches. This is not the right approach. Carbohydrates should be moved closer to the top of the pyramid, so that they form a smaller portion of our daily diets. By failing to do this, we are actually telling people to eat food that makes them sick. Another shocker on the food pyramid which really needs to be mentioned is fruit juice on the bottom shelf. Most fruit juices contain as much sugar as fizzy drinks. Fruit juice should be at the top of the pyramid with sweets and fizzy drinks.

The facts might be a little unpalatable, but it is essential that we give out accurate health information so that everyone can make informed choices. **Patients with type 2 diabetes need to know that if they don't lose weight, their life expectancy is reduced by 15 years.** They will also spend the rest of their lives on medication, and dealing with all the side-effects that come with it.

Many of my patients have managed to lose weight, reverse their type 2 diabetes and maintain their weight loss. But all of these people came to me privately. How is it possible that we cannot make the system I offer to private patients available to public patients too? It could improve so many people's quality of life, improve their prognosis and save them from the very serious complications associated with type 2 diabetes, including amputations, reduced eyesight to the point of blindness, very painful nerve damage that is resistant to painkillers, kidney damage requiring dialysis, oozing leg ulcers, chronic skin infections and bacterial infections. And improving their quality of life would also reduce the strain on our health service, taking a huge number of people off waiting lists and out of hospital beds, which would be a good outcome for everyone.

Clearly, we are not putting enough emphasis on primary healthcare and preventive medicine in our approach to type 2 diabetes. **The best, first and foremost treatment is weight loss and a healthy diet – medication should always be a last resort.**

In my experience, people who are properly motivated and properly educated don't put the weight back on. Instead of offering pills to reduce symptoms and manage the disease, we need to work hard to empower people, inspire confidence in themselves and support them to make the hard changes needed to lose weight, reverse their type 2 diabetes and enjoy the many other benefits weight loss and a healthy lifestyle can bring.

# Case Studies

## Joan Delaney
*Age 69 | Weight loss: 8.7kg*
*(1 stone 5lb)*

**Joan's story is an example of TOFI (thin outside, fat inside), but it's also an important lesson in how we should never blindly trust healthcare professionals. It is essential to remember that we ourselves are the most important member of our healthcare team. We have the ultimate say and responsibility – plus we are the ones who have to live with the consequences. This case serves as a reminder to health professionals to follow prescription guidelines instead of giving out pharmaceuticals like Smarties. After weight loss and dietary change has failed, *only then* start the patient on Metformin (Glucophage). Like many others, Joan wasn't given the chance, the right advice or the support to do that.**

*Joan went to see her GP in April 2015. She was suffering from stomach pain, vomiting and a urinary tract infection. She was given tablets to help stop the vomiting and a powder for the infection. Her bloods were taken as part of her routine six-month check-up with her GP (she was on Eltroxin for an underactive thyroid). She weighed 60kg (9st 7lb) and her doctor told her, 'You could do with losing some weight.' Joan typically weighed 57kg (9st).*

*This passing remark about her weight was not followed by any advice. Two weeks later,*

Joan went back to see her GP because she was still experiencing some vomiting. Her GP advised that her blood test results from the previous visit showed that her 'bloods were up'. There was no explanation of what was meant by this, and another blood test was performed. Joan did not get a call back from the GP with results, so she contacted them herself five weeks later. She was asked to come in and when she did, her GP told her she had 'borderline diabetes' and should lose some weight. Again, no advice, information or explanation was given – on how to lose weight or on diabetes. The next day the nurse called to tell Joan to start recording her blood sugars. She went back to her GP's clinic and the nurse showed her how to do this. A few weeks later, Joan went back with blood sugar readings and the nurse had a prescription ready to give her for Glucophage 750mg (twice a day). Weight loss, exercise and a new dietary regime were not recommended at this stage, although they had been previously mentioned. The pharmacological treatment for diabetes should only be introduced when dietary management and exercise have not resulted in adequate glycaemic control.

After starting on Glucophage, Joan started waking up at night and not sleeping well. Her home glucose readings were very erratic, and the medication did not seem to change her morning sugar readings. After two weeks, Joan got in touch with the GP's nurse and told her that she was getting quite anxious and was walking around her house with a feeling of panic and was possibly 'hyperventilating'. The nurse told her to try breathing in and out of a brown paper bag to help with the hyperventilation. Joan tried this for nearly two weeks, but by that stage she was at the end of her tether. The GP's nurse organised for Joan to go to St Patrick's Hospital on 19 September 2015.

Joan was assessed and was booked in with **acute anxiety**. She asked about her blood sugars and Glucophage, and the doctor said she would do blood tests and a glucose tolerance test.

The blood results confirmed that Joan had type 2 diabetes and while she was in hospital she was given more medication and some dietary advice. This advice was to have porridge in the morning made with milk; a brown bread sandwich with egg and salad filling and tea mid-morning; meat, potato and vegetables for lunch; another sandwich and tea in the afternoon; and a small salad with one slice of ham and vegetables for dinner. A week or two before Joan was discharged she went to see the diabetic dietitian in St Patrick's Hospital, who advised Joan to eat according to the food pyramid, gave her a small booklet, and quickly gave some advice. The whole appointment lasted about ten minutes.

The whole experience left Joan feeling anxious and worried about her health. She researched her condition herself, and that was what led her to make an appointment at my clinic in March 2017. When I first saw her, I wondered if I could I help her as she did not look even slightly overweight. She had an almost perfect waistline, but there was the possibility she might be one of those people who look and measure thin on the outside, but who are fat on the inside (TOFI), with a low personal fat threshold. I queried if she was having too many carbohydrates in her daily diet and Joan agreed with this, as she had been lighter in her younger years, prior to being diagnosed with diabetes.

At that first appointment she weighed 65kg (10st 3lb), having put on another 5kg (11lb), and at 165cm tall had a BMI of 23.8. Joan was keen to try the VLCKD and I stopped her medication for the trial period. Within a few days she started to feel better, with immediate improvement in her anxiety levels. Her glucose readings remained under 7, and three weeks later, after losing 4kg (9lb), we added some carbohydrates back into her diet and she started on Phase 3 of the diet plan. She reached a total weight loss of almost 9kg (19lb) by June 2017. Although her waistline measurements remained almost the same, her visceral fat must have reduced the insulin resistance, and this, combined with an improved diet, is the only explanation for the improvement in her home sugar readings without medication.

With Joan, it was never a question of not sticking to the diet. She gave it 100%, and still does. She really felt that the existing system here in Ireland for diabetics failed to look after her, and that if she had not taken action in looking for help, she wouldn't have got this far. We have worked closely with her to have a sensible maintenance plan whereby she has a certain amount of good carbohydrates throughout the day, with the focus on balanced protein, good fats and fibre. I am pleased to say that to date (June 2018), she has maintained her weight loss and she has officially reversed her diabetes without medication.

Joan is pleased and relieved that she kept seeking to find the help she needed. She says:

*After speaking with the clinic, I received all the information I needed to make my own decision. It sounded really good. Dr Eva took me for my first appointment on 9 March 2017, and that started the whole ball rolling. I have never looked back, I just followed what I was told to do. With further appointments with her brilliant nutritionist, I reversed the diabetes. I check my blood sugars now every three to four weeks, to keep an eye on them, and they are steady at 5.6/5.7 mmol/L, whereas in the past they were going up to 12 and 13. My current waist measurement is 80cm and I weigh 56.2kg (8st 11lb).*

Now, Joan is thin on the outside and thin on the inside!

# Miss J

*(patient wishes to remain anonymous) Age 48 | Weight loss: 12.7kg (2 stone)*

**A diagnosis of diabetes generally follows a blood test that identifies a high HbA1c level, which means that blood sugar (blood glucose) levels are elevated. A normal level is HbA1c 20–42 mmol/mol, pre-diabetic level is 42 and a reading of 48 mmol/mol means a diagnosis of diabetes. Miss J's level was 72 mmol/mol. This led to immediate medication, which in turn led to a drop in her quality of life. Her story shows that there are far better ways to achieve healthy blood glucose levels.**

*In October 2013, following routine blood tests conducted by her GP, Miss J's TSH (thyroid stimulating hormone), glucose and cholesterol levels were reported as high, as was her blood pressure. She declined medication, choosing instead to make dietary changes. She cut out processed meat, cut down on takeaways and increased her vegetable intake. Six months later her blood test was repeated and it indicated that there were no issues with her cholesterol or her thyroid, but that her glucose levels were still raised, with her HbA1c at 72 mmol/mol. Miss J's blood pressure was also slightly elevated, but it was not suggested she take any medication. Even though she had changed her diet, she was not weighed at this appointment.*

*Miss J was referred to a diabetes clinic, where she attended on 22 April 2014. She was weighed and prescribed 500mg of Glucophage twice a day. She asked the dietitian if she could forego medication and change her diet instead, but was told: 'Even if you eat lettuce all the time, you will still need medication.' She was given a leaflet about what to eat.*

*In October 2014, Miss J attended her diabetes doctor. Her HbA1c was down to 52 mmol/mol with medication. She had lost some weight and was advised to return in April 2016.*

*Miss J came to the Orsmond Clinics in September 2015 because the side-effects of the medication were impacting on her quality of life. She felt like she had a hangover every morning, had little to no energy, and experienced painful bowel problems two to three times a week, so she wanted to explore the possibility of coming off her medication.*

**When I first saw Dr Eva, she told me that I needed to lose some weight, which surprised me at the time because the diabetes clinic had told me I didn't need to lose weight and that no matter what I did, I could not change being a diabetic or needing medication. Dr Eva completely disagreed ... well, not disagreed exactly, but she told me that if I lost some weight and changed the way I eat, I could come off the medication and be off it for life, as long as I kept to the correct eating plan.**

**Dr Eva did some blood tests and told me to stop taking my medication straight away. I started on the healthy eating plan. It was fantastic to come off the medication as I was experiencing so many side-effects when taking it.**

**When I started [Dr Eva's plan], my**

*HbA1c was 52/53 on medication; it is now down to 41 with no medication. I'm not on medication now and I've lost nearly two stone in weight. I feel absolutely fantastic. I have a lot more energy and I can do a lot more walking. I am much happier now than I was because I don't feel sluggish anymore.*

*Now when I look back, I think going to Dr Eva was the best thing I've done to understand the way food reacts in my body. I think that if there was more information out there as to what exactly we should be eating at a younger age, especially for children and teenagers, it might prevent a lot of diabetes in the future.*

# John Dalton
## Age 67 | Weight loss: 50kg (8 stone)

**John was a perfect example of how a lack of information can lead to a medical condition becoming life-threatening. While John had received a diagnosis of type 2 diabetes, no one had ever suggested to him that being overweight could be the cause – and that he needed to lose weight, and fast. Once he was armed with the right information, however, he proved to have an admirable well of self-discipline to draw on. He is living proof that weight loss and weight management can reverse type 2 diabetes.**

John Dalton was diagnosed with type 2 diabetes in 1996. When he first came to see me in 2011, I told him he was a dead man walking. I know that sounds awful, but I made my calculations based on facts: the average Irish man lives until 78 years of age; John was aged 66; and type 2 diabetes takes 15 years off your life expectancy, so John had already outlived an average type 2 diabetic Irish man!

Indeed, John himself had felt like that when he was started on insulin in 2008 – it had felt like a life sentence. His blood glucose levels were not being sufficiently controlled by oral diabetic medications any more and, even more upsetting, he had to start injecting insulin. Even with insulin, his morning fasting glucose was at times as high as 11, with HbA1c at 83 mmol/mol (9.7%). He was also taking medication for blood pressure and cholesterol, as well as aspirin, a combination typical to most type 2 diabetics. It felt like a steep downward slope into ill health, until he decided to try a different approach:

*I just by accident, I suppose, found an ad for Dr Eva on the back page of the parish news leaflet. I got my daughter to ring and she made an appointment for the following Tuesday in Dr Eva's south Dublin clinic. So the first thing Dr Eva did was weigh me. She asked me what weight I was and I said I was probably 24 stone. She said, 'You're 165 kilos, which is 26 stone.' So it shocked me a little bit and I took it from there. She made me come back two days later for a weigh-in. I said there was no point weighing me after two days, but she insisted. Two days later I was down two kilos, which was very encouraging.*

*Every week I was weighed and got the diet plan for the week and because of the scepticism at home, I was more determined to stick to the plan than ever. I had tried numerous diets over the years and I would lose a stone or two and then in a couple of weeks I would have it back on again.*

*By Christmas I was down five stone, which was huge! Everyone started to notice me and some people even said, 'I hope there's not something wrong with you?' I said, 'I'm actually feeling great.'*

*I was diagnosed with type 2 diabetes about 15 years ago, and when I came to see Dr Eva, it was more the weight loss I suppose I was thinking of rather than my* diabetes, because I really didn't realise how much they were related. In 2011, when I came to see Dr Eva, my HbA1c (which is the three-monthly average of my blood levels), was 11-something, which is high, even though I was on insulin and tablets.

Eva put me on Phase 1 of the VLCKD plan of her programme. As I lost the weight on the plan I was gradually able to get the insulin levels reduced and by Christmas she decided I could go off the insulin altogether. Well, I suppose apart from the bother of doing it, it was the inconvenience of bringing the injection with you to every function you go to and having to strip off and give a prod of the needle. That's a great relief to be off the insulin, which I thought would never happen, and it's great that I lost the weight. I have heaps of energy. I'm back doing vegetable growing out in my back garden every day, in the sun. I do a lot of walking now as well. I am well able to walk now, but before I would always postpone it or find some excuse not to go for a walk. Now I have bundles of energy and I'm going stronger than I was maybe 30 years ago. I was actually really delighted because I really thought I was on a life sentence with the insulin. You know, it was something I thought would never be possible. I was delighted!

John has been off insulin for seven years and has maintained the 8 stone weight loss.

# Peggy Cheevers
*Age 65 | Weight loss: 5.4kg (12lb)*

Peggy was not a typical case, in that she wasn't overweight prior to developing type 2 diabetes. She felt well and wasn't prepared for the diagnosis. And she wasn't prepared for the rollercoaster of medications she was then told to embark on, which had a huge impact on her life. She is a good example of how pressing for information and not taking 'No' for an answer can lead to a far better outcome and a healthier life.

A routine GP check-up in late 2016 led to a shock diagnosis for Peggy; she was told she had type 2 diabetes. She was feeling fine before the appointment and was expecting every-thing to be okay. She remembers that her blood sugar reading on the day was 8.8. Prior to the diagnosis, Peggy was not taking any medication. After diagnosis, she was immedi-ately started on Synjardy (a combination of two drugs, for blood sugar), Atorvastatin (for cholesterol) and Ramipril (for blood pressure).

Peggy felt very unwell after starting these medications. The following week she returned to her GP to discuss how poorly she was feeling. The GP reduced the dosage of Synjardy. Peggy continued to feel unwell and returned again to her GP. This time, she was told that she needed to continue taking the tablets and that there was no other option.

Peggy attended a university diabetes clinic in February. She spent a few hours at the clinic, during which time she met a doctor who told her she could reverse her diabetes with exercise, but did not give her any details. She also met another woman (possibly a nurse) who said there was no way she could reverse her diabetes. Eventually, Peggy met with the consultant endocrinologist, who added another Synjardy tablet as well as Trajenta to her medication list. Peggy was told that she was doing well, but needed to reduce her HbA1c levels and blood sugar levels more quickly, hence the additional medication. In relation to Trajenta, the doctor told Peggy that he often received a round of applause at conferences when he announced that he uses this drug. Peggy was not impressed and felt uneasy about this comment. She received her sugar-reading kit at the clinic and felt that this was the main reason she was referred to the diabetes clinic in the first place.

Peggy continued to feel unwell due to the side-effects of the medications. She kept wondering if her diet wasn't as good as it could be and if this could be the reason she had developed diabetes. Then a friend of hers saw me on TV, speaking about reversing diabetes. She told Peggy, who contacted the clinic straight away:

**I got my first appointment to visit Dr Eva's clinic in May 2017. Dr Eva explained all about diabetes, how it affects the body and how it could be reversed. Being in education all my life, this was the first time I understood what was happening and how I could try to reverse it. Afterwards I came home with pep in my step. I dropped my diabetes tablets in the bin and vowed to follow Dr Eva's VLCK diet. I will not say that it was easy, but I'm quite a strong-willed person so I proceeded to follow the diet rigidly for four months.**

**I found an almost immediate drop in blood sugar levels, so this was the catalyst to continue. I never had a very sweet tooth, but I loved bread and of course didn't realise it contained sugar. I visited Dr Eva's clinic on a regular basis to monitor my blood sugar levels, my general progress and my weight loss. My husband Eamonn and I began to think differently about food shopping and I walked my dog Lucky every day to keep fit.**

**After three months on the VLCK diet I visited my own GP to get my bloods tested. Not only were my blood results wonderful, but my GP also stopped my blood pressure medication. This was the real proof that diabetes can be reversed without medication. Now, one year later, I'm a changed person. I eat a balanced diet with only an occasional treat, like a slice of bread or a scone, but without sweets. I'm always aware of maintaining my correct weight and this is a small price to pay for a diabetes-free lifestyle. I feel wonderful, having lost the excess weight, and will always be grateful to my friend Bernie who suggested that I contact Dr Eva. There's one lovely added benefit when you lose weight and that's shopping for new clothes, which is something I adore!**

# James Kelly
*Age 50 | Weight loss: 32kg (5 stone)*

**James's story is inspirational because it shows that you can turn things around, that you have the power to make changes and make a big and lasting difference. He was on a downward slide into weight gain and increasing medication, and he felt powerless to take control. But given the right help and support, he turned everything around and began climbing the steep hill back up to good health. He did it one step at a time, and his story proves that you can do it too!**

*Farmer James Kelly arrived at University Hospital Galway with a referral from his doctor to investigate his continually rising blood cholesterol levels. He left the hospital later that day with a diagnosis of type 2 diabetes and a prescription for three medications. It was the start of a difficult period in his life as he struggled to come to terms with his condition.*

*James admits that he was 'absolutely shocked' by the diagnosis and felt 'a bit down over it'. He was, after all, only 47 years old and was heading home with a 'big box of medication for a disease I didn't really understand'. At that time, he was at his heaviest weight ever, weighing almost 19 stone (around 120kg). On foot of his diagnosis, James made some changes to his diet and started going to the gym. He lost some weight and noticed an improvement in his blood glucose readings as a result.*

*A few years later, on one of his regular check-ups with his GP, his blood pressure and cholesterol medication were doubled. That was a real wake-up call for James. He began to look at the future: if this is where he was in terms of his health at age 50, where would he be at 60? How many types of medication and how much medication would he be taking then?*

*Through a friend he heard about my clinic and decided to explore an alternative route. His first appointment was in November 2016. At that first appointment, James weighed 17 stone and had a BMI of 36.8, which put him in the Obese Class II category on the overweight and obesity scale. He was taking medication for type 2 diabetes, for high blood pressure and high cholesterol, and was also on aspirin. His HbA1c was 72 mmol/mol (9.2%) despite his diabetic medication. He wasn't feeling good, and it was getting him down:*

***I was diagnosed with type 2 diabetes at only 47 years of age, my weight was increasing along with the amount of medication I was taking. I had tried many diets before which did not work for me and my lifestyle.***

***I attended Dr Eva's clinic in November 2016 and I haven't looked back. It has changed my lifestyle and attitude towards food and exercise completely. At 50 years of age I was struggling to climb up and down from my tractor, daily jobs on the farm became exhausting, I felt as if I had no energy or enthusiasm.***

Dr Eva weighed me during my first visit, and put me on a low-calorie ketogenic diet, which I was determined to stick to. I found the diet really suited my lifestyle as a busy farmer. The clinic schooled me on organisational tips like cooking my soups in advance and planning my meals, which was most definitely the key to my success.

After just five months on the diet I felt like a new man. I had lost nearly five stone and could hop up and down from my tractor with ease. I felt energised after doing my farm work and felt motivated and enthusiastic towards exercise and food preparation. I bought my first three-piece suit in years, which I couldn't have imagined in such a short space of time!

It is great to feel healthier and fitter, but the most important part of the whole experience is that I am no longer taking any medication and that has given me a new lease of life.

I received phenomenal support from my wife, kids and family, which really gave me the confidence to succeed!

When he returned to hospital for a check-up in April 2017, weighing almost five stone lighter and having completely turned his health around, the doctors, nurses and consultants were astounded by James's success. He received their congratulations and encouragement with a warning that now he had lost the weight, he had to keep it off!

Most important, the chief benefit James is enjoying due to this amazing weight loss is the reversal of his type 2 diabetes and the normalising of his blood pressure and cholesterol, which has resulted in him coming off all his medication. His HbA1c is now at 34 (5.3%) with no medication, and his once continually rising cholesterol is now only 3.7. The significant improvement James has experienced in his quality of life is all the motivation he needs to continue.

# Tom Treacy
*Age 65 | Weight loss: 13.6kg (2st 2lb)*

**Tom's story involved a complicated medical history and a suite of medications, all with a different focus and proposed outcome. He is an excellent example of polypharma and how a patient can get into a rut of medications, with new ones being added on an ongoing basis as new problems are identified. The patient in this scenario can end up feeling like a medical experiment themselves, like a pin cushion, with no control over what's happening to them. This was the situation Tom found himself in, and he was lucky to find the right help to pull him out of this rut and into better health.**

*Tom first came to the clinic in December 2016. He was 65 years of age with a very complicated medical history. His personal goal was to improve his glucose control, with the aim of reversing his type 2 diabetes that had been diagnosed 12 years earlier.*

*He was taking Eucreas (combination drug of Metformin and vildagliptin) to help reduce his blood sugar levels. Like many diabetics, he was also on aspirin, on a statin for cholesterol, and on two different antihypertensive medications for controlling his blood pressure. Tom was also using several other medications to control seizures, and to treat rheumatoid arthritis, gout and prostate. In addition to all this, he was on Nexium (to control stomach acid), which is often given to people who are taking this level of medication.*

*This level of continuous medication, otherwise referred to as polypharma, can have a serious effect on kidney function. In older patients, this 'drug-induced nephrotoxicity' can account for over 65% of acute kidney failure. With type 2 diabetes, poorly controlled blood sugars can also cause damage to the kidneys, but in Tom's case several of his medications could be linked to kidney damage.*

*Tom was in a serious situation, his health was nose-diving, and he felt powerless to do anything about it. It was a frightening and difficult time for him.*

**In 2005 I went to a funeral and met a man I had not seen for a while and he asked me how I was feeling. I said I felt good. He said, 'If you don't mind me saying, I don't think you look good! I think you should get yourself checked out.' I felt surprised, so the next day I rang my doctor and went for a check-up. So I got all of my bloods done and he rang me a few days later, saying he suspected diabetes. I felt scared as it was something I did not want to get, but a few days later I had the tests repeated and received a letter confirming that I had type 2 diabetes.**

**My doctor told me to avoid deep-fried and fatty foods and to lose weight. The idea was to try the diet approach before starting medication. After two weeks I went back and my blood tests had improved, but not enough. The tests were**

repeated again after a month and my bloods still had not improved sufficiently, so I was started on medication: Gluco-phage twice a day. I started taking this medication when I was diagnosed in 2005 and went on to take it until 2012.

In 2011 I was not feeling well. My usual GP had retired and I changed to a different GP. The GP believed the problems related to my diabetes and thought it was organ failure. I felt really frightened. He did some blood tests and after two days he told me that I had kidney failure and my whole system was poisoned by the urine. I knew there was something incredibly wrong because I was so sick that I felt like I was dying. He started me on medication and arranged for me to meet with him every morning. He took bloods every morning and after five days he was not happy and changed my medication again. This worked better and after a number of months I felt better, but my kidneys still weren't the same as I had to get up a number of times every night to go to the toilet.

Later in 2011 I developed cellulitis on my left leg. I was hospitalised with a very high temperature. My leg was totally black from my ankle to hip, and it had burst in three different places. My blood sugars were very high (over 20) and as a consequence I was put on insulin. I was taken off insulin after ten days and switched to Eucreas, which I continued taking until January 2017.

In 2015 I had a seizure. From a brain scan they discovered I had had two mini-strokes, so I was prescribed Kappra.

Then I saw an old friend, John Dalton, on TV with Dr Eva. He had reversed his diabetes, so I decided to go to see her. I knew I was overweight, but I had never succeeded in losing the weight on my own.

After my consultation with Dr Eva I started on the VLCKD plan and she stopped my Eucreas medication. As I lost weight more of my medications were reduced or stopped. A year down the road, I am three stone lighter and my blood readings are under 5 every morning. My HbA1c is 37 mmol/mol and I feel an awful lot better and don't get tired like I used to. My blood pressure has also considerably improved since and my home sugar readings are normal.

Recently I went to see a consultant in Dublin, who I had been attending for a number of years. When I met him, I told him I was attending Dr Eva. To this he replied, 'Who is this Dr Eva?' When I explained she specialised in the reversal of type 2 diabetes, he became very tense, unhappy and seemed upset. He weighed me and discovered that I had lost a good bit of weight, so he asked me if I wanted a prescription, to which I said no. He asked if I was sure and I said, 'Yes, I am sure.' He rapidly closed his folder and said, 'I will see you in six months.' An appointment in his clinic typically costs €150, so I may not bother going back.

# Brendan Coyne
*Age 64 | Weight loss: 32kg (5 stone)*

**Brendan was only in his sixties, but he was living the life of an elderly person. He was on a long list of medications, including high doses of insulin, and he lived in fear of his condition and its side-effects. He wanted to gain control of his health, but didn't feel he was receiving the right support and information to enable him to do that. His story illustrates how the currently overburdened Irish healthcare system is unable to deliver patient-centred, individualised support to those in need, instead reaching for a 'one plan fits all' approach in order to supply quick solutions to complex problems. Brendan's experience shows just how devastating this approach can be for the patient on the receiving end of it.**

*Brendan Coyne, a 64-year-old semi-retired farmer from County Galway, came to the clinic in September 2014, having been living with type 2 diabetes for the past 12 years. Brendan had worked as a builder as a young man and was a very keen sportsman, playing Gaelic football for his local club. He was very fit and active until at the age of 27 he suffered a bad ankle break that required surgery and forced him to give up sport. After that, he found it hard to do any exercise – if he tried to run, it bothered him straight away and it wasn't improving. In the early 1980s he and his wife came back to Ireland and set up a turf-cutting business. He worked very hard and was successful, but over the years the weight started to go on and it kept creeping up. One day, someone remarked that Brendan was drinking an awful lot of water and should get checked, but he did nothing. He also ignored the heavy feeling in his legs whenever he tried to exercise. Then he read an article on diabetes in a Sunday newspaper and recognised his symptoms. A visit to his doctor revealed a blood glucose level of 28 – around six times the normal reading and a really dangerous level. He was told that he had probably had diabetes for around five years without knowing it.*

*He started on treatment for diabetes, initially only tablets, but when the sugar readings kept increasing, insulin was added. He started experiencing hypo attacks, with sugar readings less than 3.9 and full-blown hypo symptoms, such as shakes and sweating. Current medical advice in the case of dangerously low glucose readings is to immediately consume some fast-acting glucose, such as Lucozade. Hypoglycaemic attack is very dangerous, and those who have experienced it describe it as a near-death experience. These recurring attacks seriously affected Brendan's everyday quality of life, and he lived in constant fear. In response, the diabetes clinic he was attending prescribed still higher doses of insulin, in an attempt to gain better glucose control.*

*Brendan's son had called the hospital on several occasions, expressing his concern for the hypos his dad was experiencing. Finally, Brendan got an appointment to see the hospital* dietitian, who told him he needed to lose weight, but didn't give any specific advice as to how to achieve this demanding task. He was advised to include carbohydrates in all his meals in order to avoid these dangerous hypos, told to watch his portion sizes and to avoid added sugar, sweets and biscuits. Brendan left the dietitian appointment more frustrated as he felt he was already doing exactly what the dietitian had told him to do. Brendan felt he was left alone to cope with the terrible hunger attacks and the life-threatening hypos.

At this point, Brendan badly needed proper support and a new perspective on his condition. After his wife read an article about the work I was doing at my clinic, he made an appointment, and that's when we started working together.

**I was not feeling like I used to. My energy levels only allowed me to work at half-pace. I used to be an active man, but now I found myself only able to drag myself on. The terrible hunger pangs and hypoglycaemic attacks were literally like a constant shadow over my days, and it took so much out of me each time with the hypos and then the need to take Lucozade. My physical and mental wellbeing were seriously affected by these feelings.**

I was, quite frankly, alarmed at the long list of medications Brendan was on, particularly the four injections of insulin per day as well as beta blockers, hypertension medications, a diuretic and aspirin. Brendan complained of 'hunger attacks', which he described as an abnormal, terrible hunger, and he also had recurring feelings of lethargy, 'fuzzy head' and tiredness, which are all signs and symptoms of poor glucose control. His weight had crept up by 19kg (3 stone) since he was first diagnosed with diabetes, and he was now just under 120kg (19 stone). He had also gained weight since starting on insulin.

As Brendan described the history of his illness and general health, it struck me that the professional team taking care of him had given up any hope of really helping him because he was 'such a complicated case'. All they seemed able to do was to administer more and more drugs rather than doing anything constructive about his weight. As he met several risk factors for heart disease, he underwent an angiogram, and a total of five stents were inserted over time to tackle blockages (atherosclerosis). He was weighed and had his waistline measured infrequently, and he didn't feel that he was given adequate information or advice to support a proper weight-loss programme. He felt it was simply a case of adding medication to medication and hoping for the best.

Since I have personally treated patients who have had diabetes for 18 years and have seen it reversed, I felt somewhat outraged when I heard all this. I started Brendan on Phase 1 of the VLCKD, designed to minimise carbo-hydrates and sugars. I felt that his cocktail of symptoms indicated that there was a high probability that he was insulin resistant, and that weight loss would fix this. We agreed to monitor his home glucose readings and, depending on the readings, we would either reduce the insulin injections from the beginning or stop them altogether. Brendan was a little nervous about coming off insulin but as I explained to him, a moderately high blood glucose reading would be less dangerous than the hypoglycaemic episodes he was experiencing when he had the 'hunger attacks'.

At his first appointment, I carried out a full medical assessment and measured his waistline, weight, height and BMI and took his bloods. His starting HbA1c was 66, and his fasting glucose was 3.

He was on cholesterol-lowering medication, and his total cholesterol and HDL were both low; in fact his HDL was only 0.8, which in itself is considered a risk factor for cardiovascular heart disease. After only two full days on the VLCKD, Brendan had lost 2kg (4.4lb). I had kept in touch with him by phone over this time, to make sure his sugars would not rise to the alarming levels typical of a diabetic patient who has been prescribed insulin to treat a defect in insulin production. As his sugars stayed at a reasonable (high) level, I was able to reassure him that this was more an indication of insulin resistance than insulin deficit, contrary to what he had been told (diagnosed) at the hospital where he had been receiving treatment.

Brendan was surprised that although the quantity of food he could consume per day was considerably reduced, he could maintain the diet due to ketone bodies and extra proteins, which the body digests slowly, thus making him feel full for longer. He came back to see me after two days, reporting that he felt better already, with more energy. Though he found the VLCKD tough and it tested his resolve, he maintained his focus on the end goal: weight loss, improved health and a better quality of life. He had already lost weight and, best of all, his blood glucose readings were good (4.5–10), still higher than for a non-diabetic but not excessively high or low.

Over the next few weeks Brendan continued to lose weight at an impressive rate: he lost 13.9kg (2st 2.5lb) in the first four weeks, his blood sugars were consistently under 10 and his blood pressure was reduced. Brendan mentioned that before the diet he had had a swollen leg, but that the swelling had now completely gone and he felt better than he had in years – much sharper, more alert and more energetic. There was a certainly a spark in Brendan that hadn't been there the first day I met him and his enthusiasm for this new regime was great to see.

The only difference in Brendan's medication up until now had been the removal of the insulin injections from day one of the VLCKD, and a full set of blood tests was done every month to keep me up to date on how the weight loss was affecting his health biomarkers; I also kept his GP informed by regular email contact. I checked Brendan's blood pressure at his routine visits to my clinic and noticed that it was coming down consistently with the weight reduction. Brendan reported that he felt dizzy at times when he was working, and I recommended he get a 24-hour blood pressure monitor fitted. This revealed that he had moderate hypertension at times during the night, but that the daytime levels were normal.

As time went on we reviewed Brendan's diet and after two months, and a weight loss of over 22kg (3st 7lb), we introduced fruit and small amounts of regular carbohydrate foods, like porridge and lentils. At this time Brendan's

Case Studies

GP reduced his cholesterol-lowering statin medication as his blood results showed a significant reduction in his cholesterol levels to 2.2.

Christmas came and went, Brendan still continued to lose weight and feel better. He had lost a total of 31kg (5 stone) after four months and his waistline measurement was reduced, indicating that he was losing the visceral fat. He was happy on the diet and attended a consultant endocrinologist, Dr Wilma Lourens, whose opinion I greatly respect. Dr Lourens congratulated Brendan on his achievement and the 'fantastic improvement' in his general health. She suggested a change in his medication for hypertension as she noted he had orthostatic hypotension (low blood pressure when standing) and was experiencing dizzy spells at times. Brendan's own doctor agreed to reduce one of the beta blockers and soon afterwards he stopped taking them altogether and the dizzy spells stopped. Although Brendan didn't officially reverse his diabetes, he was a new man. His HbA1c level was 44 mmol/mol with 1,000 mg Glucophage only. He was not experiencing the terrifying hypos or any of the other symptoms that had been so severely limiting his quality of life.

Brendan was encouraged to introduce new foods to his diet, such as avocado, nuts and coconut milk, and to increase consumption of healthy oils and slow-releasing carbohydrates, like sweet potato and beans, to maintain steady blood sugars. He was also eating small amounts of wholemeal bread, but saw immediately how it affected his blood sugars if he overdid it on the portion size! Brendan was now eating a really good diet with plenty of vegetables, homemade soups, eggs, fish and lean meats, along with small amounts of slow-releasing or low glycaemic index (low GI) carbohydrate foods. He has maintained his weight loss and continues to reap the benefits of his new, healthier self:

**I would strongly recommend Dr Eva's expertise and motivation, as it helped me to turn my health and life around. I now enjoy the best levels of energy, fitness and health that I have had in over twenty years. The programme was not easy, but the reward is more than I could have ever hoped for. I feel very good – brilliant! I'm able to do so much more and I'm able to manage my diet, eat out and enjoy life to the full!**

# Terry Burke
*Age 70 | Weight loss: 16kg (2st 7lb)*

Terry is 70 years old, active and intent on enjoying a healthy retirement. This ambition was being hampered by various medical issues, as well as by his weight. He had tried various diets over the years, experiencing the up-and-down wave of weight gain and loss that will be wearily familiar to many dieters. The will to achieve the weight loss was there, but the supports and information were not. Terry is nothing if not persistent, though, and when he finally located the right support at my clinic, he achieved his goals and hasn't looked back!

*Terry tells his story in his own words:*

*A quick background. I recently retired as Master Marine in the Merchant Navy, a profession which was to find me as the captain of various ships, until in 2013 I took command of the MV Maersk Lamanai in South Korea, classed as a Very Large Container Ship (VLCS). My quarters were situated on J Deck, which was ten decks above the main deck and nine above the Mess decks, where we would take our main meals. On previous vessels I had commanded my quarters were on F Deck. This meant that I would regularly take the stairs before and after meals. Now, the additional four decks proved too much and I would take the elevator.*

*I already had a problem with my weight going back to 2000, when I began to suffer from pains in my knees brought on by arthritis, although I wasn't aware of the cause for some years. Being the typical male I soldiered on and put up with it until it became too intense and, in 2006, I sought medical advice. I was diagnosed with advanced arthritis and informed I would require full knee replacements. I had my first operation in May 2007.*

*Unfortunately, I suffered complications and instead of healing in 12 weeks it would be six months before I would be passed fit for sea duty.*

*I tried several diets to keep the weight down, but inevitably once I returned to sea it would balloon back up. At times I found myself wishing I could get back to 14 stone, which was my weight when it all began.*

*The experience with the first knee replacement put me off having the same procedure on my right knee, until I reached the stage when the injections had little effect. So in 2010 I bit the bullet and had the second op. This was a great success and I was fit within three months. I did not help myself, however, and eventually in 2014 I tipped the scales at 17 stone.*

*This [weight gain] was accompanied by several medical problems, including snoring and sleep apnoea, breathlessness and the need to double the strength of my blood pressure tablets. (I had had hypertension since 2004.) I was already prone* to high cholesterol and my doctor had put me on statins to combat this.

In February 2017 my ship spent two weeks in dry dock, and this involved visiting the dock bottom several times a day to inspect work being carried out. The increase in physical activity improved my wellbeing and I lost some weight, but not a lot. When I went on leave in April I had my bloods taken by the practitioner's nurse. This was a precaution as both my late mother and elder brother suffered from type 2 diabetes. The following week, I was informed I, too, had type 2 diabetes. My GP immediately put me on Gluco-phage and Diamicron. The latter had an adverse effect, including a couple of episodes of hypoglycaemia, and I stopped taking it within a week.

Although registered as a type 2 diabetic, getting access to the various services proved difficult, especially as I was due to return to the ship for my final voyage in July. It was at this time I saw an advert in the Irish Times promoting a workshop by Dr Eva titled 'Type 2 Diabetes, Curse or Reverse' to be held in Moran's Red Cow Hotel on Sunday 28 May, and we booked two places.

The relationship between carbohy-drates and excess glucose particularly struck me because back in 2004 I had been on the Atkins Diet and lost a consid-erable amount of weight, but in the end was not happy with the balance and came off it – and, of course, ballooned again. Dr Eva offered, to me, a much

healthier and more structured way to not only lose weight but potentially reverse [type 2 diabetes]. I enrolled and attended my first appointment the following Wednesday, 31 May. During the interval between the meeting and my appointment I used the free Eurodiet samples received at the meeting, so I had started the diet before I officially became a patient. By the Wednesday I had lost 2.2kg, so already things were looking positive.

The need for me to return to sea in early July for three months created a challenge for Dr Eva and, if truth be known, for myself, but after taking bloods and various measurements a plan was formulated and I was handed over to one of her dietitians. She formulated a dietary regime backed up with Diet Diaries and using the Eurodiet products, along with great recipes for soups and various ways to cook vegetables, which I had no problem sticking to. In addition, on Dr Eva's instructions I ceased taking the Glucophage, which meant I was totally off diabetes medication.

As somebody who enjoys cooking, it was easy for me to prepare my own meals and I got great satisfaction from the results. By sticking to the advice I managed to maintain the weight loss while on holiday in Portugal and upon rejoining my ship my first task was to examine the cook's latest Victualling Stores order and increase the amounts of fresh vegetables.

*My wife, Eithne, had been travelling with me since her retirement and during the course of the voyage she went ashore and bought clothes a size smaller for me. By the time I left in October, I needed clothes two sizes smaller. I had lost six inches off my waist, three inches from my neck and had gone from XXL to L.*

*My first clinic appointment upon my return was on 23 October and the bloods showed improvements all round. The latest measures, in early 2018, confirmed that Dr Eva has kept her promise to reverse my type 2 diabetes, for which I am extremely grateful. The positive attitude of herself and the encouragement from her staff has played a major part in keeping me motivated and on track.*

*It has been something of a personal triumph for me that I have managed to achieve the weight loss and now, as I settle into retirement, I have still a bit to lose, but not much, and we will be working on a maintenance regime in the very near future.*

## Pat Mulcahy
### Age 74 | Weight loss: 25kg (4 stone)

**When Pat Mulcahy heard the word 'impossible', he felt his fate was sealed. This was the verdict of an endocrinologist when Pat asked if there was any other way to manage his diabetes, for example, through diet. He was told it was 'impossible'. This is a bleak illustration of what happens to so many patients – their care team sees only the narrow path of medication, and refuses to look at other possibilities and options. Pat's story shows that 'impossible' can be converted into 'very possible'!**

*I first met Pat in 2014, when he came to the clinic as a last resort. He had been diagnosed with type 2 diabetes 14 years earlier, and since then his condition had deteriorated. He was on eight tablets a day and the prognosis was not good. In January, his consultant told him that the damage to his kidneys from the diabetes and the medication meant he had to start using insulin, and that he had to prepare himself to commence dialysis. This is a difficult thing for any patient to hear, and Pat was understandably upset and anxious, hoping there were other options available to him. When he asked if a medically supervised diet could help, his specialist told him that there was no way he could avoid going on insulin. When he put the same question to his endocrinologist, he was told: 'You could become the fruit and veggie guy, but it would be impossible to do that diet.' So it was impossible; not even worth trying.*

*Everyone Pat spoke to told him to stick to the medication, that there was no way out.*

*Thankfully, Pat didn't give up. In February, he made an appointment to see me and we began to work together, and he started on the VLCKD. This was the first time in 14 years of treatment that Pat had received dietary and lifestyle advice and the support to see it through. I was the first person to tell him he needed to lose weight!*

**Back in 1999 I noticed that I was thirsty all the time. A year later things had not improved and I was passing urine very frequently, up to twenty times each day. I went to my GP and he took some blood tests.**

**The result of the blood test determined that I was type 2 diabetic. After a short time I was taking 4x500mg Glucophage plus 4x30mg Diamicron. This went on for about 14 years, and by then I was attending a diabetes clinic every three months. At some stage in 2004 the specialist at the clinic informed me that the tablets were no longer working and I would need to go on insulin injections. When I asked what that would mean, he said that I would probably put on a few more stone in weight. At this time I was already 19 stone 7lb (125kg); my weight had always been around 15 stone (95kg) before my diagnosis.**

**I had read a newspaper article about Dr Eva and the reversal of type 2 diabetes. None of the medical people that I was dealing with thought it was possible, so on that note I decided to contact Dr Eva. That was the best decision I ever made. There was no**

*mention of medication, just a strict diet, under the strict supervision of Dr Eva herself and her team of nutritionists. After just three months I had lost three and a half stone and my diabetes control and bloods were much improved. I have never looked back and although my weight has increased a bit since, I can still control my blood sugars with just one tablet each day. Dr Eva for president is what I say!*

By June of that same year, not only did he no longer need to go on insulin, he had also avoided dialysis and significantly reduced his diabetic medication. So in just five months, 20 short weeks, he had achieved the 'impossible'!

Now, four years on, Pat continues to keep his diabetes under control without insulin and has avoided dialysis. While he feels it is a constant battle to keep the weight off, he keeps up the fight every day – because it's far better than the alternative!

# What is Diabetes Mellitus?

The word 'diabetes' was first recorded in 1425. It means a 'siphon', referring to the excessive urination associated with the disease. The Greek word *mellitus*, meaning 'like honey', was added in 1675 to reflect the sweet smell and taste of the person's urine. Yes, before the days of sophisticated laboratory tests, doctors tasted urine for sweetness to confirm the diagnosis!

Thankfully, times have moved on, but in reality the most recent knowledge for treatment is not being used, even in our sophisticated university hospitals here in Ireland. It is simply bad patient care and contrary to medical ethics that professionals who make life-changing decisions about the care of their patients are not required to be up to speed with the latest treatments. I know that money and resources are limited, but in this day and age when a patient goes to their doctor asking if they can either reverse their type 2 diabetes or at least reduce their medication load, they are typically told: 'There's nothing you can do; you need to take these medications for life.'

Type 2 diabetes is still being defined as a chronic progressive disease: 'chronic' meaning that you will have it forever (and will typically have already been suffering from it for quite some time, as it takes around seven years from the start of your silent symptoms to diagnosis); and 'progressive' meaning that it will only get worse with time. This may be true if no action is taken. The initial reaction from medical professionals is typically based on administering drugs and/or vague comments, such as 'You could try to be more active and clean up your diet' or 'You could try to lose some weight.' This is not very encouraging! In fact, I have looked after patients who felt they were so badly treated at the time of their diagnosis that they started experiencing acute anxiety, which in turn caused them serious problems (see Joan Delaney case study, p.11).

Whatever happened to empowering the patient to take charge of their own health? I believe that if a newly diagnosed type 2 diabetic, or someone with pre-diabetes, was treated with the same respect and care as someone who has just been diagnosed with a life-threatening condition, we wouldn't have these epidemic levels of type 2 diabetes. The 'pill for every ill' treatment is partially caused by the fact that some people want to continue living their lives the same way, without making any changes. Perhaps they see no other way, or maybe they just can't be bothered! Or is it that many doctors don't believe that a patient can make the necessary changes? As a result, prescriptions are dished out as both the patient's and the doctor's preferred choice. But even the doctors' prescription guide states that medication should be the last resort, 'if lifestyle changes have failed'.

Diabetes is a group of metabolic disorders characterised by high blood sugar. This is the result either of the body's inability to produce (enough) insulin or the body's inability to respond to insulin. There are two main types of diabetes: type 1 diabetes and type 2. If you are affected by either of them, something has gone wrong with your pancreatic function.

The pancreas, like other endocrine organs, produces hormones, which are basically just chemical messengers. When your blood sugar is low, your pancreatic alpha cells produce glucagon – a hormone. This stimulates the liver to start breaking down the stored glycogen into glucose (glycogenolysis). When blood sugar is high, your pancreatic beta cells start producing the insulin hormone, which 'tells' the cells that there is glucose available as an energy source, but also stimulates the excess glucose to be stored as glycogen and stops the breakdown of fat in adipose tissues.

## Type 1 diabetes mellitus (T1DM)

Type 1 diabetes is an autoimmune condition where the immune system destroys beta cells. Currently, there is no cure for this condition and the patient requires lifelong use of insulin. However, I disagree with the current practice of 'injecting for normal living', whereby the patient injects the amount of insulin that is required for each meal, without needing to control their carbohydrate intake in order to take less insulin! They are much more likely to gain weight with this practice, and make their health worse. Although the ketogenic diet does not suit type 1 diabetics, we have used a reduced carbohydrate weight-loss diet in my clinics (Phase 3, see p. 82), with the benefit that the person needs less insulin. A smaller insulin requirement also enables weight loss.

## Type 2 diabetes mellitus (T2DM)

This type of diabetes is characterised initially by insulin resistance, which is usually followed gradually by insulin deficiency, meaning the beta cells get exhausted and don't produce enough insulin. The beta cells of the pancreas initially produce insulin, but for some reason (not yet exactly known, but see p. 34 for more information on visceral fat and insulin) the cells of the body don't respond to it the way they used to, and glucose stays in the bloodstream instead of being used up by the cells as a source of energy. To put it simply, this makes the pancreas try to produce more insulin in the hope that the higher level of insulin will be a sufficient 'messenger', and that the cells can take in the glucose they have been told to take.

Think of it like closed doors (closed cells) that are not opening because there is just one person banging on them (insulin). The pancreas then sends more people to bang on the closed doors (more insulin). Eventually, the doors open, the glucose floods in and the blood sugar drops. The

What is Diabetes Mellitus?

abnormally high blood glucose results in the typical medical symptoms of type 2 diabetes, and the sugar readings stay abnormally high. These typical symptoms are excessive urination, thirst, tiredness, recurrent infection, e.g. urinary tract infections, thrush (vaginal and in skin folds, e.g. under breasts), sores and cuts that won't heal, and blurred vision. The high sugars are initially treated with oral hypoglycaemic medications. Due to the combination of insulin resistance getting worse, an unbalanced high-carbohydrate diet and possibly recurring viral and bacterial infections (which alone cause high blood sugars), the sugar readings climb even higher. When the current oral hypoglycaemic medications have been exhausted, the doctors reach for the last resort: insulin injections.

It is well recognised in clinical practice and research that insulin injections come with a high price, not only physically (their side-effects), but also in terms of financial costs to society. For example, John Dalton (see case study, p. 16) has saved the Irish government about €5,000 a year for over seven years by not needing insulin. Some of the worst side-effects are life-threatening hypoglycaemic attacks and weight gain, which is well presented in the case of Brendan Coyne (see case study, p. 23). If a patient is still producing some of their own insulin and it's therefore more a question of insulin resistance, and they are now injecting more insulin as a form of treatment, it makes it extremely difficult to manage their glucose control and weight, and they feel extremely

hungry. They are also risking hypoglycaemic attacks as they don't know how much insulin they actually need.

With time, the production of insulin slows down when a person has carried visceral fat for many years, and it eventually stops when the beta cells are totally exhausted under the effect of the low-grade inflammation coming from this visceral fat. This is when a type 2 diabetic is considered to have become a type 1 diabetic. (An estimated 30% of type 2 diabetics become type 1 diabetics in time.)

The medical solution presented for type 2 diabetics is drugs: drugs that make the pancreas produce more insulin, drugs that make the cells more responsive, drugs that take the excess sugar away. However, none of them solves the problem and they all cause (or at least do not stop) ongoing damage to the pancreas and side-effects to the rest of the body. Typically, half of type 2 diabetic patients need insulin injections ten years after diagnosis.

Until the 1990s, type 2 diabetes was not readily associated with obesity. It used to be differentiated from type 1 diabetes as non-insulin dependent, 'adult-onset' diabetes. There are other risk factors, including diet, genetics, sleep apnoea and age, but **the leading cause of type 2 diabetes is excess visceral fat**. With the huge increase in overweight and obesity levels worldwide, and a matching increase in type 2 diabetes over the past 20 years, what causes type 2 diabetes is now very clear. What is now also very worrying is that it is affecting much younger people, including children.

I have met so many type 2 diabetic patients who were told that they did not need to lose weight, or that it would make no difference to their condition if they did. They have been seriously misinformed! Every single one of them who subsequently changed their diet and lost weight either reversed their diabetes or significantly improved their condition. So let's not keep looking for other excuses and 'risk factors' when the cause is staring us in the face!

**Body fat**
We all need some body fat to insulate us, to prevent our organs getting damaged and to supply us with a stored form of energy for later use. The anatomical term for body fat is adipose tissue, which is made up of adipocytes, or fat cells. This tissue is mainly found around the internal organs (visceral fat) and underneath the skin (subcutaneous fat). These fat cells are sensitive to insulin and they can store fat.

But what is the link between type 2 diabetes and visceral fat? One of the simplest ways to understand visceral fat is to picture your poor pancreas covered and surrounded by fat, which suffocates its function. When this fat doesn't know where to go, it starts to infiltrate the cells, stopping the organ functioning properly, similar to a case of fatty liver. Excess fat is simply not supposed to be stored in these tissues.

The thickness of the subcutaneous (under the skin) fat increases when we consume more calories than our body needs. It shows on the outside of our bodies as general 'plumpness' and as fat around the middle. This is what we refer to as 'visible' fat. The subcutaneous layer of fat that we are able to pinch between our fingers is not the dangerous fat; however, it usually reflects the amount of visceral fat we are storing. So the more excess weight you have around your middle, the more excess visceral fat you are likely to be carrying.

Visceral fat is stored within the visceral cavity, around organs such as the stomach, intestines, kidneys, pancreas and liver. Because visceral fat is situated deep in the visceral cavity, it can go completely unnoticed because it's not visible to the naked eye. In fact, there are people within a normal body mass index (BMI) range who have dangerous levels of excess visceral fat. This explains why some 'thin-to-the-eye' people get type 2 diabetes.

The technical term TOFI (thin outside, fat inside) would apply to many of my patients (see the case studies of Miss J, p. 14, and Joan Delaney, p. 11). In some cases, the only way to discover this visceral fat is by taking a picture of the inside of the abdomen using an MRI or DEXA scan, but this is not commonly done.

An easy, cheap and very practical way of estimating the amount of visceral fat you might have is to take a waistline measurement. **Your waistline should not measure more than half your height (in centimetres).** So if I am 160cm tall, for example, half of which is 80cm, then ideally my waistline should be no more than 80cm. If my waistline is 86cm, it indicates that I have an extra 6cm around my waistline. Each extra centimetre represents 1kg (2.2lb), so if I have an extra 6cm around my waist, I am 6kg (13.2lb) overweight. In this case it would be advisable for me to lose 6kg.

**How type 1 and type 2 diabetes are diagnosed and how wrong diagnoses are possible**

Diagnoses of type 1 and type 2 diabetes are usually done clinically, which means that patients are diagnosed according to the symptoms they present with at the time they seek medical attention. Although type 2 diabetics can in time become type 1 (insulin-dependent) diabetics, most type 1 diabetics are diagnosed at a young age. They are typically very sick at the time of seeking help, presenting with symptoms such as unplanned weight loss, increased thirst and a frequent need to urinate. Often they present to medical care in ketoacidosis, requiring ICU treatment, which immediately makes doctors think of type 1 diabetes.

They may also have been experiencing unusual weakness and hunger. It was generally thought that if a patient had these symptoms, they would be diagnosed with type 1 diabetes and started on a lifetime of insulin.

The difficulty in differentiating between a type 1 and a type 2 diabetes diagnosis is that some of the symptoms can be identical. However, there are tests that are used to help make a correct diagnosis. If the level of ketones in the blood or urine is tested, they may be high – but they can be high for different reasons. For example, a small amount of ketones will be present in the urine of someone who has not eaten for several hours, or higher amounts will be present in someone who is following a ketogenic diet. Typically, though, high levels of ketones are an indication that someone with diabetes generally is deficient in insulin and needs insulin treatment.

I need to clarify a common misunderstanding between two words that sound very similar: ketosis and diabetic ketoacidosis (DKA). DKA is marked by extreme accumulation of ketone bodies. It is very rare in type 2 diabetics and luckily not common in controlled type 1 diabetics. During this accumulation, the blood pH drops, the blood becomes too acidic and the blood sugars remain high. DKA requires immediate medical attention. Ketosis, on the other hand, is merely a marker that you are producing some ketones (by-products of burning fat). You can be producing these ketones naturally if you are following a low-carbohydrate diet or if you are fasting. The body can operate perfectly well in a state of ketosis, and it is only in situations where insulin levels are very low or there is no insulin production (type 1 diabetes) that a state of ketoacidosis occurs. In (nutritional) ketosis, you do not produce enough ketones for them to cause ketoacidosis.

A normal ketone-induced diet (ketogenic diet) will result in ketone body concentrations of around 3 millimolar, whereas ketoacidosis occurs at concentrations of around 15–20 millimolar. In comparison, starvation-induced ketosis has ketone levels in the range of 3–6 millimolar. So, if you stick to a sensible ketogenic diet, have insulin production (or are insulin resistant) but are not type 1 diabetic (with no insulin production), you are not at risk of ketoacidosis.

Type 1 diabetics typically present with antibodies against the islet cells (beta cells), and these can be measured. This is not the case in all type 1 diabetics, but if these antibodies are present in the bloodstream, it is very likely the person has type 1 diabetes. Another blood test can measure C-peptide, which is part of the insulin molecule. If C-peptide is found in the blood, it means that some insulin is being produced and it's more likely that the person has type 2 diabetes.

In clinical practice I have, unfortunately, seen many type 2 diabetics who have been on several diabetic tablets for years before they have finally been started on insulin. As you can see in the section on pharmacotherapy (see p. 53), Diamicron–sulphony-lurea, for example, is known to slowly kill the beta cells of the pancreas. If a person has been on that particular medication for years and has also carried a lot of excess visceral fat, these things together will have caused some permanent damage that I cannot predict at the beginning of their diet. This is another reason why I may have to take several blood tests and the patient must remain under close medical supervision (especially at the beginning of the diet), in order to determine the changes needed in their medicines. Thankfully, the human body has an amazing capacity to heal itself. I have seen many incredible cases of healing when a person loses that excess fat, reverses their insulin resistance and their beta cells kick back into action.

You can see how easy it is to make a wrong diagnosis, especially if it's based only on symptoms and a busy hospital or medical practice does not carry out further laboratory tests. It just takes a doctor under pressure making one quick decision to help a sick patient with high sugar readings and ketone bodies for the patient to receive the wrong diagnosis. Afterwards, nobody questions the diagnosis. It is accepted, and the patient is told this condition is lifelong and treatment gets under way. The poor patient does not know any different.

This sort of mistake is particularly common for overweight patients who had insulin resistance due to their excess weight and who, after a bad infection (e.g. a head cold), suffered a complication such as pneumonia. A bad infection typically sends glucose

What is Diabetes Mellitus?

readings through the roof and if the patient was feeling very sick and not eating a lot, that is the logical reason why the ketone bodies were present in their body. Can you get the picture?

Years ago, I had the pleasure of helping a gentleman called Brendan Coyne (see case study, p. 23). He was on high doses of insulin, but was suffering from many low sugar-level attacks (hypos). His son was seriously concerned about his father and brought him to see me. He was insulin resistant, but was just given more and more insulin to bring down his sugar readings. His condition didn't improve until he changed his diet and started on VLCKD, lost weight and came off all his insulin. Pumping the body with more insulin is not always the right decision, especially if you are insulin resistant. And sometimes it makes things worse, as Brendan's story shows.

Insulin is a hormone that is naturally produced in the pancreas and its function is to control the level of glucose in the blood. To be more specific, it's produced by the beta cells in the islets of Langerhans, which is in the pancreas. When we consume carbohydrates, our glucose levels rise, and this releases insulin into the bloodstream. This response to an increase in blood glucose typically takes about ten minutes. In people with diabetes, however, these cells are either attacked and destroyed by the immune system (type 1 diabetes), or they are unable to produce a sufficient amount of insulin for successful blood sugar control (late stage type 2 diabetes). This is why diabetics are treated with insulin – to create the right response to glucose.

The downside of insulin treatment is that it raises the risk of hypoglycaemia, can cause weight gain, can pose a problem for those who are uncomfortable with self-injecting, and can affect the ability to drive, which could be a major problem for some people, especially if their livelihood depends on driving (www.diabetes.co.uk/driving-and-hypoglycaemia.html). So you can see that while there can be medical reasons for choosing insulin, it has its drawbacks – not least the fact that it promotes weight gain, which is the cause of the problem in the first place!

### BMI vs waist measurement

Your excess weight is the obvious first cause of your diabetes that you can do something about. Many overweight people don't realise that they are overweight, and it doesn't help that most doctors don't weigh their patients. In fact, weighing should be as routine as checking your blood pressure. People who are overweight often compare themselves to other, bigger people and feel that they are not as bad as them, or that their weight is 'not bad enough' to cause diabetes. I find that people usually have a personal opinion about what they think is a healthy weight for them. Sometimes this is based on a memory of when they felt and looked well – for example, when they were wearing a certain size of clothing.

As a result, when treating patients we can sometimes run into a heated conversation about what the ideal weight actually should be. I have to explain to people that this is not based on my personal opinion, but that I can calculate it by using a measuring tape. It is very simple: your waistline measurement is the most accurate and reliable way to track your weight because your waistline should be no more than half your height in centimetres.

I'll use the example from earlier to illustrate this again: if I am 160cm tall, my waistline should be no more than 80cm, or half my height. So if my waist measures 86cm, I am 6kg (13.2lb) overweight, and I must lose those extra kilos. If I am 160cm tall and weigh 63kg (9st 13lb), I would still have a 'healthy' Body Mass Index (BMI) of 24.6. But if I carry even just 2cm excess on my waistline, this excess weight could mean that I am exactly as discussed above: thin on the outside, fat on the inside (TOFI).

It is clear that we need to be careful about just measuring people's BMI. The healthy BMI range is very wide, from 18.5 to 24.9. A BMI of 22 is typically considered to be an ideal, healthy BMI. This is best illustrated with an example. For my height, my ideal weight is 57kg (8st 9lb). But within the healthy BMI range this could vary by 16.5kg (2st 5lb), from 48kg (7st 5lb) to 64.5kg (10st 1lb). At 57kg (BMI=22), my waist measurement would be around 81cm, but at 64kg my waist would be 88cm. At 88cm, I would have a visible tummy bulge and clearly this would be indicative of fat around the middle (visceral fat).

Sometimes people who have a normal BMI get diabetes. It seems to come down to the individual, and also perhaps because everyone has their own personal fat threshold (Taylor & Holman, 2015). These normal weight people are typically told by their doctors and healthcare professionals that they got diabetes because it's genetic, therefore there is nothing they can do about it. That's that – just accept it.

I have met so many type 2 diabetes patients who were told that they did not need to lose weight or that it would make no difference to their condition if they did. Clearly this is not the case! Every single one of them who subsequently changed their diet and lost weight has either reversed their diabetes or significantly improved their condition. This was the case with both Miss J and Peggy Cheevers (see p. 14 and p. 17), who were told that even if they ate only lettuce leaves and lost weight, they could not reverse their 'chronic progressive disease'.

When I first saw Miss J, I was unsure whether or not I would be able to help her. But the moment I measured her waistline and noted that it was more than half of her height, and she told me that her lowest weight in her adult years was 8 stone (50.8kg), I realised there was a big chance that her diabetes 'lived' in the extra 10cm around her waistline. As we now know, an extra 10cm equals an extra 10kg (1st 5lb).

And, in fact, that turned out to be the case. After seeing Miss J's case and other similar cases, I have come to trust the waistline measurement even more.

If you happen to be one of those people with a pre-disposition for type 2 diabetes, even a small amount of excess weight and visceral fat could be enough to affect the beta cells and insulin production. For the 'lucky' ones, most of whom probably have better insulin production, it appears that their systems can tolerate a higher amount of visceral fat before diabetes sets in.

**Chronic inflammation**

In the past, excess fat was thought to be just a reserve for energy, but it has since been discovered that visceral fat produces hormones, which are biologically active substances. Due to this hormone production, visceral fat can be described as an endocrine organ in its own right. These hormones are inflammatory in nature – in other words, they seem to create a low grade of inflammation throughout the body. Although a certain amount of inflammation is vital for our body's healing processes, it is when the inflammation gets out of control that our bodies almost get 'irritated' inside. This is why visceral fat has such a bad reputation, but what we can do to reduce it is seldom discussed.

This inflammation is not only related to insulin resistance, but is also now recognised as a driving force in the increasing levels of

cancer, and it may be an underlying cause of other chronic diseases, including heart disease. All this information is out there, and I strongly encourage every reader to look into this themselves (a good starting point is www.medicalnewstoday.com, and you can also talk to your GP for information and advice), so that you can make educated decisions about your own health.

Not everyone with excess body weight develops type 2 diabetes, so why is it that some people escape it and others can't? Could it be possible that medication, which is clearly intended to give a better quality of life and a longer life, actually causes the disease that you have?

The problem, as we have seen earlier, is that medical professionals tend to treat the symptoms, not the cause. As a result, there seems to be one plan for everyone, even though we are all individuals and very different from one another. In symptom-led medicine, once the symptom disappears, for example glucose control improves with medication, the problem is considered to be resolved. But that doesn't answer the key question: why did it come to be a problem in the first place? High glucose levels are not due to a 'deficiency' of Metformin any more than a headache is caused by lack of paracetamol.

Having said all this, there are a number of health professionals who are willing to question the standard mode of practice, even if it sometimes means putting their own jobs at risk. The highly respected UK-based cardiologist Dr Aseem Malhotra believes that insulin resistance is the number one cause of heart attack, the precursor to type 2 diabetes and also independently linked to high blood pressure, dementia and cancer.

The reasons why little is being done to treat type 2 diabetes correctly is baffling. Is it just lack of information, or misinformation, or simple denial of what the real problem is? Take cigarette smoking as an example. It took over 50 years after the first links were made between smoking and lung cancer in the *British Medical Journal* for effective regulations to be introduced that reduced smoking rates. This was because the tobacco industry successfully adopted a corporate strategy of planting doubt about the contention that cigarettes were harmful, confusing the public, outright denial and even buying the loyalty of scientists. The extent of that denial went so far that the CEOs of every major tobacco firm went in front of the US Congress in 1994 and swore under oath that they did not believe nicotine was addictive and that smoking caused lung cancer. Thankfully, we now know better.

I have not met any type 2 diabetics who received any explanation regarding the serious side-effects of their prescribed medications. I feel terribly sad and angry when people say, 'The doctor put me on this and it's only 5mg a day.' Would 5mg of arsenic over a long period of time go unnoticed?

This might sound very extreme, but as far as I'm concerned if the problem can be solved with diet and lifestyle changes, that is what the prescription should be.

### Why do some people get type 2 diabetes and others don't?

It appears that some people are more prone to develop type 2 diabetes than others, and while we don't know exactly why this is, there are a few hypotheses that researchers are busy exploring. The following are a few different factors that have been blamed. (Please note that I have not listed these in order of importance.)

**Age** is considered a risk factor for type 2 diabetes. Our organs and general system functioning weakens as we age and our body becomes fragile and less resistant. However, I still personally believe that this often goes hand-in-hand with excess weight because people typically put on weight as they get older. Many blame 'middle-age spread', which is caused by hormonal changes, among other things, but again this is just an excuse. With age we often become less active, which leads to extra calorie accumulation.

**Bad diet**, specifically **high sugar intake**, has been blamed, even in the absence of weight gain. High sugar intake leads to excessive insulin production, which could be the reason for insulin exhaustion and resistance, but the exact mechanism is not yet known.

**Low activity levels** and a 'couch potato' lifestyle. Muscle is the only part of our body that doesn't need insulin to utilise sugar, and this could be the reason why low activity levels require more insulin. The list of benefits of exercise is long and convincing, from improved circulation to reduced insulin resistance and more balanced hormone production.

Another risk factor that is not often discussed is **metabolic programming**. A lot has been written about it recently in the scientific literature, but it doesn't seem to have filtered down. It is considered one of the major causes of the increasing levels of obesity and many other chronic conditions like type 2 diabetes. When nutritional stress, such as overfeeding during an important period of early development, permanently changes the body's physiology and metabolism, it's called metabolic programming. The importance of adequate nutrient intake during pregnancy is well recognised. Overnutrition is now considered a form of malnutrition. When an expectant mother consumes excess nutrients, i.e. energy and food beyond the normal requirements for her own and the growing baby's needs, it's an oversupply relative to the amount needed for normal growth, development and metabolism. All of this ties in with an increased risk of adult-onset ill health.

If you are in your fifties or older, it is unlikely that your mother was obese while expecting you because very few people were obese fifty years ago. If you are younger or have a daughter planning to start a family, it's important to be aware of metabolic programming. You should ask yourself if there is a possibility that your current lifestyle, diet and weight may not only affect your future health, but that of your offspring.

## Type 3 diabetes (or Alzheimer's disease)

It has been suggested that Alzheimer's disease should be renamed type 3 diabetes because, as recent studies have found, insulin resistance can also develop in the brain. Post-mortem reviews of people with Alzheimer's found that clumps of protein, called beta-amyloid plaques, had formed between the brain cells. These same beta-amyloid deposits are found in the pancreas of many people with type 2 diabetes. It is thought that these deposits may block communication pathways within the brain, hence contributing to the development of Alzheimer's.

Researchers have also found that a number of signs linked to diabetes are present in Alzheimer's, which is one of the most common forms of dementia, affecting an estimated 55,000 people in Ireland, with that number growing all the time. As we already know, high blood sugars cause inflammation throughout the body and brain. This chronic inflammation has been linked with two brain changes typical of Alzheimer's disease. (For more information, see www.diabetesselfmanagement.com/blog/type-3-diabetes-symptoms/.)

Another possible contributor to the development of Alzheimer's is 'tau tangles'. These are twisted-up proteins that form within nerve cells and interfere with cell function. While it is unknown what causes this nerve damage, studies carried out at Brown University in Pennsylvania indicate that insulin resistance, the core of type 2 diabetes, may deprive brain cells of the glucose they need to function, thus causing damage.

Studies show that approximately half of people with type 2 diabetes will go on to develop Alzheimer's in their lifetime. In other words, type 2 diabetics have a 50–65% higher risk of developing the disease than non-diabetics. Those with high cholesterol or high blood pressure are also at greater risk.

## Diabetes and cancer

According to Dr Mary Ryan, a consultant physician and endocrinologist, 'In the care of the diabetic patient, note that their cancer risk should be taken into consideration when choosing anti-diabetic therapy.' This is because diabetics are twice as likely to get cancer of the liver, pancreas and uterine lining. Their risk of colon, breast and bladder cancer is also a shocking 20–50% higher than non-diabetics, although there does not seem to be any higher risk for other cancers, such as lung cancer.

So where is the connection? There are cells growing abnormally in our bodies constantly, but we have very sophisticated systems in place to stop them developing into cancer cells. Cancer cells basically do not 'listen' to all the signals that would normally prevent them growing out of control, and once the cancer cells start developing, they don't listen to the signals that would normally kill them. What recent research has found is that high blood sugar and high insulin levels – both found in patients with type 2 diabetes – seem to interfere with the processes that would normally prevent uncontrolled cell growth and the death of 'out-of-control' cells.

According to Dr Mary Ryan, 'Diabetes induces insulin, insulin-like growth factors, oestrogen, cytokines and other growth factors. The interaction of these hormonal factors is likely involved in cancer promotion as most of these hormonal factors play a role in carcinogenesis (the formation of cancer).' Too much insulin (hyperinsulinaemia), high blood pressure (hypertension), fat-induced chronic inflammation, obesity and diet all play a role in the biological link between diabetes and cancer. Not only that, but as all diabetes medication is involved one way or another in the control of blood sugar, there are different pathways that could promote cancer development, depending on your medication.

## Diabetes and sleep apnoea

Obstructive sleep apnoea (OSA), also known as 'the silent epidemic', is a serious medical condition and probably more common than you think. In Ireland, 6,500–7,500 people were diagnosed with OSA in 2016 (Irish Sleep Apnoea Trust). This might be just the tip of the iceberg, however, as EU medical researchers suggest there are possibly around 100,000 people in Ireland affected by it, whose symptoms range from mild to severe.

When a person with OSA is asleep, soft tissue at the back of the throat collapses and closes temporarily, which causes a blockage that prevents regular breathing. This interruption of deep sleep interferes with the body's metabolism, making it a key risk in the development of diabetes. Scientific research has shown that people who are overweight (BMI 25–29) and obese (BMI 30+) have a higher risk of developing OSA because when the level of fat in the throat increases, the size of the airway decreases. This is a danger particularly when you are sleeping because it is during these hours that the muscle in the throat relaxes, and the fatty tissue effectively builds up in the airway and blocks it.

The apnoea-hypopnoea index (AHI) increases by around 30% with every 10% weight gain. A neck circumference test can be helpful in determining whether someone is at high risk for OSA. For men, the high-risk measurement is 43cm (17 inches) or higher; for women, it's 40cm (16 inches) or higher. The symptoms that signal apnoea are snoring, excessive sleepiness during the day and 'brain fog'. If you suspect that you have sleep apnoea, visit your GP, who may refer you to a sleep specialist.

## Understanding the terminology around blood sugar levels

We have encountered the term HbA1c, particularly in the Case Studies section, and it's an important term to understand. It stands for glycated haemoglobin, haemoglobin A1c. Haemoglobin is the oxygen-carrying protein in red blood cells. This becomes bonded with glucose (sugar) in the bloodstream. This bonding is called glycation. The higher a person's blood glucose levels have been, the higher the number of red blood cells that will have become glycated, and therefore the higher their HbA1c level. This is why it's an effective test of blood sugar levels.

As the red blood cells exist in the body for around three months, the HbA1c test reflects the person's blood glucose over a longer period – approximately for the previous 8–12 weeks – compared to only measuring blood glucose levels, which measures the blood sugar at the time the test blood was drawn (which changes quickly and all the time depending on exercise, stress and diet).

The World Health Organisation (WHO) suggests the diagnostic guidelines for diabetes on the next page.

| HbA1c level (mmol/mol) | HbA1c level as percentage | Status |
| --- | --- | --- |
| *Below 42* | 6.0% | Non-diabetic |
| *Between 42 and 47* | 6.0–6.4% | Impaired glucose regulation (IGR) or pre-diabetes (it is common practice to start patients on Metformin when HbA1c is 42 or over) |
| *48 or higher* | 6.5% | Type 2 diabetes |
| *Below 53* | 7% | Type 2 diabetic in good glucose control. Above this level indicates poor control |

*Note: the way we report the test changed a few years ago from % to mmol/mol, but many (myself included) are still used to and prefer to use %.*

If your HbA1c is 48 or over, you are diagnosed as diabetic. If your HbA1c test returns a reading of 42–47 mmol/mol (6.0–6.4%), that indicates pre-diabetes. Your doctor should suggest weight loss if your waistline exceeds half your height in centimetres. The response to this diagnosis should be diet change and an assessment of your overall lifestyle. While nothing can be guaranteed in medicine, I can confidently say that at this level, **pre-diabetes can be reversed**. This is the moment to react decisively and stop the disease developing into full-blown type 2 diabetes.

### Why is HbA1c important?

HbA1c really is the king of glucose monitoring because it gives an overall better idea of what your average blood sugar levels have been over the past 12 weeks or so. This is incredibly important and useful information in tackling diabetes. When your HbA1c has dropped under 42 mmol/mol, nobody is interested in your daily glucose readings any more. I always say to my patients that I prefer their HbA1c to be under 40 mmol/mol (e.g. 39), as 42 is too close to bad! But in reality, once your HbA1c is 41 mmol/mol, you are no longer pre-diabetic and daily home glucose readings can be stopped.

There are huge benefits that come with lowering HbA1c levels. Studies have shown that if type 1 and type 2 diabetics reduce their HbA1c levels by 1% (or 11 mmol/mol), they cut their risk of dying within five years by 50% (European Association for the Study of Diabetes (EASD), September 2012). They also reduce the risk of developing microvascular complications by up to 25%. This includes retinopathy, neuropathy and diabetic nephropathy (kidney disease).

Furthermore, in the case of type 2 diabetics, a 1% reduction in HbA1c levels can reduce the risk of suffering cataracts (by 19%), heart failure (16%), and amputation or death due to peripheral vascular disease (43%).

### How is HbA1c tested?

The test itself is very simple. A blood sample is taken from the patient and sent to the lab for testing.

While the HbA1c test is usually reliable, there are some limitations to its accuracy. For example, people with forms of anaemia may not have sufficient haemoglobin for the test to be accurate and may need to have a fructosamine test instead. Being pregnant or having an uncommon form of haemoglobin (known as a haemoglobin variant) can also return an inaccurate HbA1c, while readings can also be affected by short-term issues such as illness, as this can cause a temporary rise in blood glucose.

Due to the way the HbA1c test measures blood sugar, if you have higher blood sugar levels in the weeks leading up to the test, this will have a greater impact on your result than your glucose levels two to three months before the test.

# The Role of Smoking and Alcohol

A healthy lifestyle benefits all of us, but for those with diabetes there are even more compelling reasons to address bad habits, such as smoking, alcohol consumption and inactivity.

## Smoking

I am most definitely anti-smoking. It is a dangerously unhealthy habit and you must break it and give up smoking for good. This applies whether you are pre-diabetic, diabetic or not diabetic at all. There is no benefit whatsoever of smoking tobacco, it only brings disadvantages and hazards. If you do have type 2 diabetes, the dangers are even more pressing.

Diabetes is a vascular disease, which means that long-term health consequences arise from the damage and changes caused by the combined effect of fatty deposits in the walls of blood vessels and hardening of the blood vessels. Smoking causes similar damage to the walls of the arteries, so you can easily understand why smoking and diabetes together strengthen the negative effects of both and speed up the damaging effects.

Over time the fatty deposits restrict blood flow and cause micro- and macro-vascular (small and big vessel) problems in the heart, brain and kidneys. They also cause peripheral artery disease (PAD), which is when blood vessels in the extremities (especially the legs) become blocked or narrowed due to these fat deposits. The reduced blood flow to all the extremities, such as your legs, feet, male sexual organs and lower back, can cause many problems:

- chronic lower back pain
- erectile dysfunction, which is a clearly visible sexual dysfunction in men
- decreased libido and difficulty reaching orgasm in women, which can often be mistaken for 'bad luck', but in reality are the results of the small vessels becoming blocked, which affects not only the nerve function but also the sensation
- peripheral artery disease (PAD), which presents with a variety of symptoms, such as leg cramps or pale and blue-tinged legs due to poor circulation, feeling numb or cold in the lower legs, sores or ulcers with infections, and hair loss on the legs, which typically only men notice
- generally extended healing times for any injuries.

Smoking and diabetes both increase the risk of heart disease in very similar ways, so when combined they greatly exacerbate the chances of suffering a heart-related condition, such as a heart attack or stroke.

## Alcohol

We all know that alcohol can cause serious health problems, and that it is also not good for us from a weight-loss perspective. Did you know that 1g of alcohol contains 7kcal? This is second only to fat, which contains 9kcal/g. Protein and carbohydrates contain only 4kcal/g. This means that one small bottle of wine (187ml), which has about 20g alcohol, amounts to 140kcal. When you add in the sugar and other content, the calories shoot up even higher. And there is little nutritional value: drinking alcohol is simply drinking calories!

Alcohol cannot be taken at all in Phases 1 and 2 of the VLCKD because it drops blood sugars and causes carbohydrate cravings. I see a lot of type 2 diabetic patients with high gamma-glutamyl transferase (GGT) levels, which are used to detect possible liver damage, and they are commonly asked by their GP if they drink a lot of alcohol. You would need to drink massive amounts of alcohol to increase your GGT levels. This increase is more often due to fat in the liver. When visceral fat doesn't know where else to go, it infiltrates the inside of the liver. When it reaches its limit in the liver, it infiltrates other organs. A fatty liver is very serious as it eventually leads to cirrhosis (hardening of the liver).

I understand that cutting out alcohol or reducing your intake to a minimum is easier said than done. I love white wine, and I always have to fight the devil sitting on my shoulder to avoid it, but it's better to try to only drink in company. Most people tell me that when they haven't drunk alcohol for three days, they realise it was just due to habit that they used to sit down in the evenings with a drink.

Many diabetics have taken nightcaps of alcohol with the intention of lowering morning blood sugar levels (because they've noticed it had this effect), but remember that your morning sugars won't rise when you have got rid of the fat in your middle and reversed your diabetes!

When you reach the maintenance phase of the diet, there is nothing wrong with having a small glass of wine or a unit of other alcohol in the evening. It's all about moderation and enjoying a small amount, which is the right attitude to take with alcohol.

Flavonoids, which are chemical compounds found in colourful fruits and vegetables, are present in small amounts in wine and other types of alcohol, and because of this the idea has emerged that a glass of wine is beneficial to diabetics. This is incorrect. The amount of flavonoids contained in wine is not enough to justify the claim. The beneficial effect of a small quantity of alcohol every day actually comes from the anti-aggregation of our platelets: stopping the platelets from sticking together might have a beneficial effect in the prevention of heart attacks and strokes. That effect is not limited to wine – it comes from any type of alcohol.

Of course, with alcohol comes the all too well-known carbohydrate cravings. Not only does alcohol itself contain calories, it makes us much more likely to stray from a diet plan, and then makes it much more difficult to get back on track again. So, like anything else, we need balance when it comes to alcohol.

A unit of alcohol is 10ml of pure alcohol (ethanol). Simply saying that a unit of alcohol is a small (100ml) glass of wine or a half pint of beer is very misleading because it does not take into consideration the huge differences in strengths and measures of wines, beers and spirits.

The number of units of alcohol in a drink depends on:

- how strong it is
- the volume of the drink.

The number of units of alcohol can be determined by multiplying the volume of the drink (in litres) by its percentage alcohol (by volume) (ABV).

A 500ml can of beer at 4.3% ABV contains:

**0.5 x 4.3 = 2.15 units of alcohol**

On average a bottle of wine (750ml) at 13% contains ten units of alcohol.

**(0.75 x 13 = 9.8 units)**

A few examples:

- A small (100ml) glass of wine at 9% is 1 unit.
- A large glass (250ml) contains 3.0 units.
- A 35.5ml pub measure (in Ireland) of vodka or whiskey at 40% is 1.5 units.
- A small (50ml) glass of sherry, fortified wine or cream liqueur (approximately 20% ABV) is about 1 unit.

There are seven calories per gram of alcohol. This is second only to fat, at nine calories per gram. A few examples are:

- Pint of Fosters – 193kcal
- Pint of draught Guinness – 210kcal
- Pint of Heineken – 227kcal
- Gin and tonic – 120kcal
- Smirnoff Ice – 228kcal
- Jack Daniels, single (25ml) – 64kcal
- White wine, dry (175ml) – 116kcal
- Smirnoff Red (20ml) – 44kcal
- Champagne (175ml) – 133kcal
- Martini, single (50ml) – 70kcal

So, a simple warning: alcohol equals calories!

# Driving and Diabetes

Can you drive when you have type 2 diabetes? Yes, you can – it is not an issue. However, you do need to ensure that your blood glucose levels are steady and within normal levels, otherwise your ability to focus – and even your eyesight – could be affected. For this reason, it's particularly important to check your glucose levels before driving if you are on any medication that has the potential side-effect of increasing the risk of hypoglycaemia. Insulin, sulphonylureas and prandial glucose regulators are the class of drugs you need to be particularly careful of, or any drug that has a combination ingredient of this in it.

If a person suffers from hypoglycaemia, they become drowsy or dizzy and need to get their blood sugars under control immediately. During a hypo attack, a person loses consciousness. Hypo is a life-threatening situation and this is obviously a huge risk when driving. It has shocked me several times, when discussing medication and lifestyle with my patients, to find out that they were completely unaware that a drug they had been using for years (e.g. Diamicron, or a drug that was a combination of sulphonylurea and Metformin) posed a potential risk of hypoglycaemia. As a result of not knowing this, they had never checked their blood sugars before driving.

I have met some patients who had been prescribed the sulphonylurea class of drug and been on them for years without even knowing *how* to check their blood glucose or having the equipment (blood glucose monitor) to do so. This is serious, and it is the type of situation that should not happen in a well-managed healthcare system. You should always carefully read the medication information leaflet included in the drug package. Every drug contains this information leaflet. Unfortunately, it is very common for people not to read it. Also, the pharmacist and the doctor prescribing the drug should have informed the patient about this. The patient is potentially risking not only their own life but also others' lives if they drive in these conditions!

If a person gets warning signs of hypoglycaemia while driving, it is important to stop driving as soon as it is safe to do so. In fact, a person is committing an offence if they continue to drive after becoming aware that they have signs of hypoglycaemia or that they are feeling unwell (RSA, 2017). The signs of hypoglycaemia are:

- sweating
- trembling or shakiness
- weakness
- hunger
- increasing or fast pulse or palpitations
- feeling anxious/anxiety
- tingling sensation in the lips.

More severe symptoms include:

- slurred speech
- difficulty concentrating
- feeling confused
- irrational behaviour.

The Road Safety Authority (RSA) has guidelines (2017, see www.rsa.ie) for drivers who have diabetes or who are being treated with insulin. Some of these guidelines include the following.

- Always carry a glucose monitor and blood glucose strips. Make sure the meter displays the correct date. Check blood glucose before driving and every two hours while driving.
- Always have personal ID that highlights that you have diabetes in case of an accident.
- Always stop driving if you develop hypoglycaemia. If you experience hypoglycaemia, turn off the engine and remove the keys. Get out of the driver's seat and do not drive for at least 45 minutes after the blood glucose level has returned to normal.
- Keep a supply of fast-acting carbohydrates in case of emergency.
- Make sure to take rest breaks and to stop for meals and snacks regularly.
- Avoid alcohol.

If you have ever experienced any of these symptoms while driving, or if you are surprised to hear of this potential risk, please talk to your GP or diabetic clinic to get clear, solid information about what to do and what not to do. It's very important that you are well informed so that you can drive safely at all times.

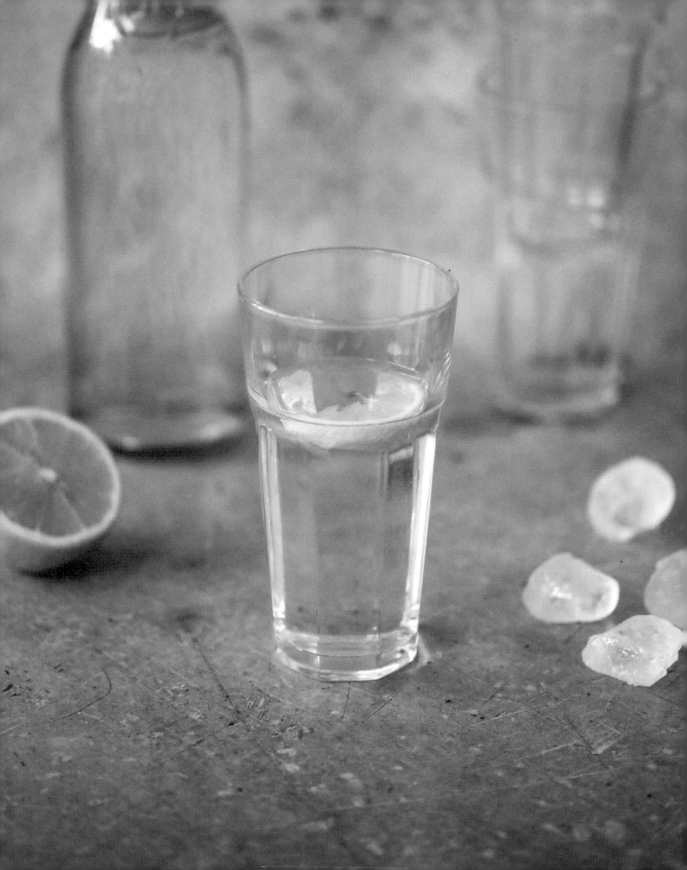

# Diabetes Medication and its Side-Effects

The following section has been written for people who have either decided that changing their lifestyle and diet is not a priority for them at this point or who don't feel that, under their current circumstances, they are able to put in the functional changes required to reverse their type 2 diabetes. The table on pp. 56–59 lists the most commonly used prescription drugs in the treatment of type 2 diabetes and their potential side-effects and suitability for VLCKD. The purpose is to encourage patients to know their medications and the currently accepted treatment protocol.

While the conventional approach to the treatment of type 2 diabetes in Ireland does not yet really recognise (with a few exceptions) that the reversal of diabetes is possible, earlier International Diabetes Federation (IDF) treatment guidelines advised that pharmacological treatment of type 2 diabetes should only start when lifestyle change with weight loss, diet and exercise have failed.

However, under the IDF's new guidelines, which came out in 2017, it is up to the primary care physician to either immediately start the patient on medication along with lifestyle changes, or to delay the start of medication for up to six months if they think that the patient is able to reach acceptable glucose control with lifestyle change alone. So far, I have observed through my patients' experiences that many doctors don't believe that their patients will make the necessary lifestyle changes, and just start their patients on medication without even offering them the lifestyle change option.

There are some progressive GPs out there who take time to advise their patient on the importance of changing their lifestyle and to lose weight prior to introducing medication. Unfortunately, this is rare. Typically when type 2 diabetes is diagnosed, a patient is prescribed a cocktail of drugs to treat not only increasing sugar levels but also high blood pressure (ACE inhibitor) and cholesterol (statin) and anti-platelet therapy with aspirin.

Advice in this section is based on IDF clinical practice recommendations for managing type 2 diabetes in primary care. I have also added additional information from my own clinical experience – what I have learned from my patients – regarding side-effects, drug interactions and their suitability on a VLCKD, to give you more knowledge to enable you to make an informed choice and not just leave the decisions and management of the disease to your healthcare professionals.

While I believe that most people can reverse their type 2 diabetes, I acknowledge that some need pharmacotherapy. Equipping yourself with more knowledge will motivate you to look after yourself with minimum medication and help you, with your healthcare team, to choose the right drug combination. The lower the medication load, obviously, the fewer the side-effects. It goes without saying that every pharmacotherapy comes with side-effects. It's a question of weighing up the benefits against the disadvantages.

When researching the different side-effects of diabetic drugs listed in the table below, information varied hugely between sources. I found that cancer was a reported side-effect for a certain class of drugs (DPP-4 inhibitors), but when trying to follow up on these reports I made contact with the pharmaceutical company Merck. The representative I spoke with told me they have no records outlining such side-effects, as these were US FDA (Food and Drug Administration) report findings and are therefore not recorded in the EU, even though it is the same drug. Looking into side-effects is very complex. For example, you have to consider whether the link with cancer is coincidental or not, since all patients with type 2 diabetes mellitus are twice as likely to get cancer in the liver, pancreas and uterine lining anyway. It is always going to be difficult to evaluate how much the risk of cancer is due to the drugs themselves. The main emphasis of this table is to make you question whether taking these drugs is

worth increasing the risk you already have of diseases such as cancer. You, and your lifestyle, are the most important determinant of your health outcome.

Pharmacotherapy of type 2 diabetes is governed by international guidelines set by the IDF and NICE (the UK's National Institute for Health and Care Excellence), and all healthcare providers should not only master them, but also follow them in clinical practice. Unfortunately I don't see this happening in practice; for example, I regularly see patients with Metformin dosage exceeding the maximum amount.

My biggest concern with pharmacological treatment is the possible occurrence of hypoglycaemia. I have met several patients over the years who were on drugs that can cause hypoglycaemia without knowing about it! Of all of the different types of glucose-lowering oral medication, the sulphonylureas and glibenclamides/glyburides are associated with the greatest risk of hypoglycaemia. Clearly, insulin injections pose the highest risk of potential hypoglycaemia.

The ideal glucose control for type 2 diabetics is HbA1c under 53 mmol/mol (7%). With this level, the long-term medical complications of type 2 diabetes are believed to be progressing at their minimum speed. The *IDF Clinical Practice Recommendations for Managing Type 2 Diabetes in Primary Care* says that 'Although the risk of diabetic complications decreases with lower values of HbA1c down to the normal range, the main concern in decreasing HbA1c to a target far below 7% (53mmol/mol) is doing more harm than benefit with aggressive treatments that induce hypoglycaemia and weight gain.'

Metformin (with Metformin hydrochloride) is always the first line of treatment choice as monotherapy for the management of type 2 diabetes.

According to the guidelines, a second medication (doctors usually call it second agent) is added if after a minimum of 3–6 months the glucose control (HbA1c) is not acceptable. Although the baseline HbA1c for starting on a combination therapy varies by as much as 58–75 mmol/mol (7.5% to 9%), it is up to the prescribing physician to make a call on starting the dual therapy.

The second drug added is typically sulpho-nylurea (typical brand name Diamicron). The side-effect profile consists of the dreaded hypoglycaemia and weight gain, and even worse, the seldom-mentioned beta cell degeneration (usually called beta cell exhaustion). But as more drug classes have become available in recent years, the main motivating factor being to create a drug that would help in weight loss, the new SGLT2 (sodium-glucose co-transporter-2) inhibitors have become more commonly used because they have been associated with modest weight loss. It all sounds great until you look at the side-effects. I would not agree with using this class of drug – the price is very high in terms of their severe potential side-effect profile.

When one drug does not do the job, a second is added. When the glucose is still not lowered enough, guess what? A third drug is added. Is this really a sensible solution to cure this disease? All these pharmacological ingredients have side-effects that can damage the kidneys, liver and the whole physiological system. When a person is treated with three oral diabetic medications, clearly the cumulative side-effects are huge.

How many drugs are you taking? You might only be taking one tablet, but some medication combines two drugs in the same tablet. Be aware of this, as well as the dosage of each of the drugs you are taking – not just the tablet. There are so many combinations of Metformin and DPP4-inhibitors (e.g. Janumet), Metformin and SGLT2 inhibitors (e.g. Synjardy), Metformin and sulphonylurea that one pharmacist I spoke to called it a 'minefield'. When drugs are combined in this way it is obviously difficult to tell which component of the drug is causing the side-effects.

The information in this table is based on my research and my clinical experience. As with any medical issue, you should speak to your own doctor about any concerns you have and seek a second opinion if you are unhappy with your current treatment or the side-effects of any medication you are taking. Bear in mind that the names of medicines often change, so this list is not exhaustive.

Diabetes Medication and its Side-Effects

| TRADE NAME | HOW IT WORKS | BACKGROUND | SIDE-EFFECTS |
|---|---|---|---|
| Glucophage or Metformin Mylan | Delays absorption of glucose from intestines; reduces glucose released in bloodstream; helps cells respond to insulin; makes body utilise insulin better in the muscles. Does not pose a risk of hypos. Good at lowering HbA1c. Is often used in treating PCOS. | Metformin has been used for over 40 years but was only approved by the FDA in 2007 due to concerns. | Nausea, vomiting, upset stomach or diarrhoea. Headaches, muscle pain, weakness, flatulence. Vitamin B2 deficiency. Tiredness. Taste disturbance. |
| Diamicron MR, Diaclide MR and Amaryl (sulphonylureas) | Lowers blood glucose levels by forcing the pancreas to stimulate more insulin. Improves overall glucose control. Lowers HbA1c effectively. | First developed in 1956; typically used as a second drug prescribed in addition to Metformin. But due to serious side-effects, DPP4 and SGLT2 inhibitors are now the preferred option. | Slowly exhausts and ultimately results in total loss of beta cell function. Weight gain, hypoglycaemia, skin disorders (itchiness, redness), swelling of the throat, causing difficulty breathing. |
| Forxiga, Invokana, Jardiance (SGLT2 inhibitors) | Increases the excretion of sugar in the urine; inhibits reabsorption of glucose in the kidneys. | In July 2011, the FDA recommended against approval until more data was made available. In January 2014, the FDA approved Dapagliflozin (Forxiga) for glycaemic control along with diet and exercise. It was approved in the EU in 2012. | Hypoglycaemia may affect 1 in 10 people; this figure is even higher when the drug is taken in combination with other diabetic medication. Urinary tract infections and genital infections (thrush). Linked to acute pancreatitis. Increased risk of bladder cancer. Risk of lower limb amputations. Renal side effects. Frequent urination. |

| CONTRAINDICATIONS | OBSERVATIONS | ADVICE TO MEDICAL PRACTITIONERS |
|---|---|---|
| Should not be prescribed for anybody with reduced liver or kidney function (creatinine > 150 umol/L). Cardiac or respiratory failure, recent heart attack, shock. Alcoholism. Pregnant or breast-feeding women. | Maximum dose should be 2000mg per day, but I often see 3000mg, which is counter-productive as the side-effects far outweight the benefits. Nega-tively affects renal system and stomach. | People who are on VLCKD should have this medication reduced or even stopped – I have had a few patients whose blood sugars went too low. Metformin usually causes gastrointestinal discomfort. It is beneficial to stop this medication when starting VLCKD in order to minimise flatulence. |
| Should not be prescribed in con-junction with medications to treat thrush infections. Breastfeeding or pregnant women. People who are overweight or obese. Type 1 diabetes. Severe renal or hepatic insufficiency. Not to be used in conjunction with alcohol or phenylbutazone-based drugs. | In my opinion, this is a drug class that should be avoided at all cost due to the damage it causes to the beta cells. The longer you have been taking these, the less likely you are to reverse your type 2 diabetes. | This medication must be stopped when starting a VLCKD as it could lead to hypos. The VLCKD diet is low in carbohydrates, which can be dangerous if combined with taking the drug. |
| Moderate to severe renal impair-ment. Type 1 diabetes or for the treatment of diabetic ketoacidosis. Loop diuretics. Patients with a history of low blood pressure or other cardiovascular diseases. Do not take if you are galactose intolerant or have low salt levels in your body. Not to be used in conjunction with drugs containing Pioglitazone. | I am personally totally against the use of this type of drug. In my opinion, the cons by far outweigh the pros. While I have seen some patients lose weight, the strain this drug puts on the kidneys, and the potential side-effect profile, make it too risky. I believe that the mechanism of action causes what I think of as 'renal bulimia'. | This medication must be stopped when starting a VLCKD as there is a high risk of hypoglycaemia. |

Diabetes Medication and its Side-Effects

| TRADE NAME | HOW IT WORKS | BACKGROUND | SIDE-EFFECTS |
|---|---|---|---|
| Bydureon, Byetta, Victoza and Trulicity (incretin mimetics) | Increases production of insulin. Supresses secretion of glucagon. | Byetta was the first incretin mimetic drug to be approved for treating type 2 diabetes. | Hypoglycaemia is very common. Severe allergic reaction and bowel obstruction. People are usually very unwell, especially when they start taking the medication. Nausea, headaches, vomiting, diarrhoea. Loss of appetite, indigestion, acid reflux and constipation. |
| Trajenta and Januvia (DPP-4 inhibitors) | Increase the levels of incretin hormones and thus how much insulin is released from the pancreas. | Approved in 2011 by the FDA, to be used together with diet and exercise. | Pancreatitis. Hypoglycaemia. Gastrointestinal problems (nausea, diarrhoea and stomach pain). Flu-like symptoms and skin reactions. Serious allergic reactions. Dizziness and drowsiness have been reported. |
| Novorapid, Levemir, Lantus, Humalog, Tresiba (insulin) | Novorapid is short-acting. Humalog works quicker than normal human insulin because the insulin molecule has been changed slightly. It is designed to more closely mimic the body's own natural output in response to eating a meal. Levemir is a modern insulin with a long and steady blood sugar-lowering effect 3–4 hours after injecting. Tresiba is long-lasting and only needs to be injected once a day. Modern insulin products are improved versions of human insulin. | Humalog was FDA-approved in June 1996. Levemir was first approved by FDA in 2005. | Hypoglycaemia. Weight gain is very common. Injection site reactions such as localised erythema, pain, pruritus, urticaria, oedema and inflammation. |

| CONTRAINDICATIONS | OBSERVATIONS | ADVICE TO MEDICAL PRACTITIONERS |
|---|---|---|
| Type 1 diabetics. Diabetic keto-acidosis. Severe liver disease. On dialysis. Symptoms of pancreatitis. Severe stomach or gut problems, or IBS. Heart disease. | I am personally totally against the use of this type of drug as the cons far outweigh the pros. While some of my patients reported losing a small amount of weight while on the drug, they stopped taking it as they felt so unwell on it. | This medication must be stopped when starting a VLCKD as there is a high risk of hypoglycaemia. |
| Type 1 diabetics. Treatment of diabetic ketoacidosis. Alcohol should not be taken. Pregnant or breastfeeding women, women planning to become pregnant. | Often prescribed when patients cannot take Metformin. In my opinion it is not worth the risk of the side-effects. The risk of hypoglycaemia is increased when taken in combination with other diabetic medication. | Combine with a healthy diet. You can take this while doing a VLCKD but it is not necessary. |
| If you think hypoglycaemia (low blood sugar) is starting. | Should be used as a last resort as type 2 diabetes mellitus results from insulin resistance and giving more insulin won't rectify the problem; you are just adding more insulin to an insulin-resistant body. Should only be used by type 2 diabetics with little or no beta cell function. | Either stop or significantly reduce to, for example, a third of the dose, when doing a VLCKD. This needs to be monitored closely with the patient, especially in the first few weeks. |

Diabetes Medication and its Side-Effects

## A note on Warfarin

Warfarin (Coumadin) is typically prescribed as a blood thinner (anti-coagulant) in order to reduce the formation of blood clots in veins and arteries in high-risk patients, e.g. patients suffering from atrial fibrillation. The main aim of Warfarin is to prevent arterial and venous thrombosis and stroke. As with all pharmaceutical drugs, it comes with risks. The predominant risk with Warfarin is bleeding, which has the potential to cause significant morbidity or mortality if not monitored closely. For many patients, however, the increased risk of clot formation or stroke means that the risk of harm from Warfarin therapy is acceptable. When you reduce your risk factor profile by losing weight and changing your lifestyle, you should have a serious re-evaluation with your doctor to establish whether you can stop taking Warfarin. It can be hard initially to get the dosage of this drug right, and medical professionals may even recommend against any new dietary regimen, such as changing your diet.

Warfarin blocks vitamin K, which facilitates the function of several proteins, including those that are responsible for blood clot formation. As green leafy vegetables contain abundant amounts of vitamin K, if your diet contains a lot of vitamin K, this will cancel out the effect of Warfarin. In other words, if you eat a lot of green leafy vegetables, you are wasting your time taking Warfarin and unnecessarily putting your body at risk of side-effects without gaining the benefits.

Green vegetables are also a major source of other important nutrients. From a dietary point of view, they should form the biggest part of what you eat because you get so few calories and carbohydrates from large servings that are full of fibre, and they keep you fuller for longer. The key to getting the nutritional benefits from vitamin K without it affecting the use of Warfarin is to take in a consistent amount of it every day. A good rule of thumb is to have 100ml (half a cup) of cooked green vegetables with each of your main meals, e.g. half a cup of spinach with your breakfast, a soup with cauliflower and broccoli for lunch and for dinner a stir-fry made with (peeled) courgette, white cabbage and green French beans or green pepper or a full cup of green salad leaves.

You can eat as much of the following vegetables as you like while on Warfarin: tomato, cucumber, artichoke, courgette (peeled), red cabbage, red pepper, turnip, aubergine, mushrooms, cauliflower. (Beetroot, onions, pumpkin and carrot are also okay, but not on the VLCKD due to their higher carbohydrate content.)

# Very Low-Calorie Ketogenic Diet (VLCKD) Explained

I always tell my patients that there are many ways to get to Rome. It's not necessarily *how* you lose excess weight; the most important thing is that you make the effort to lose it! This might sound surprising because so much has been written about the supposed 'adverse effects' of unhealthy and fad diets. Some may be true; but others are judged on the basis that they don't follow the food pyramid!

The recommended weight-loss method presented on many government websites as the only healthy way to lose weight is through a low-fat, reduced-calorie diet following the conventional food pyramid with the aim of slow weight loss of about 0.5kg (1.1lb) per week. The idea behind this is that if you lose weight slowly, you are more likely to modify your behaviour in the long term and therefore will find it easier to maintain your weight loss. Slow weight loss does work for some people, but in reality most people lose motivation if they don't start seeing results quickly and soon go back to their old habits, and I speak from 15 years of clinical experience treating overweight and obesity.

That is where the VLCKD steps in: rapid weight loss that gets results and gets you motivated. It is a total break from eating habits based on the traditional food pyramid, and once you have lost the weight and stopped eating all those excess carbohydrates, you can put the effort into learning new eating habits and sustainable weight control.

There is no one diet that suits everyone, and this is why my clinics offer individualised approaches to losing weight. When you first come to see me, I gather information about you that helps me determine the most suitable diet for you, one that fits your needs and goals.

A person with only a few pounds around the waist to shift will notice a 1lb weight loss very quickly. An obese person, by contrast, will hardly notice anything until the weight loss is substantial because the weight is spread throughout their body.

Generally speaking, people with a lot of excess, unhealthy weight are also those who need to make the biggest changes to their diet and therefore they need the biggest motivation. If they don't see any results, they are more likely to give up, especially if after making so many changes nothing seems to be happening. On the other hand, if the weight loss is quick, the motivation is higher and it doesn't seem like an unachievable task any more!

It is not only about what people see on the scales. Weight loss comes with several other benefits, such as improved home glucose readings, lower blood pressure (with less or no medication required!), more energy, less bloating, fewer aches and pains, freer breathing (this is one of the first things that improves), the feeling of being back in control and generally feeling better. People notice these benefits much more quickly when the weight loss is faster and they are not feeling as many negative effects of their excess weight.

In contrast, it is more difficult to lose weight when your calorie requirements are smaller. While VLCKDs are traditionally not recommended for people with a BMI less than 24, I have found it to be effective for people requiring a small amount of weight loss. You will see from Peggy's and Miss J's case studies (p. 17 and p. 14) that even a small amount of excess weight can cause type 2 diabetes – and losing less than 1 stone (6.3kg) can reverse the condition.

There is a difference between the requirements of someone who wants to lose weight when they are metabolically healthy and have not yet experienced medical complications, and someone who has had complications, especially something as serious as type 2 diabetes, and has been prescribed medication to treat it. While you should be able to reverse your diabetes even if you lose excess weight slowly, my experience – and plenty of research – suggests that there's something very beneficial about

quick initial weight loss through the VLCKD method.

**Please note:** All type 2 diabetics on glucose-controlling medication should only attempt to lose weight under medical supervision. Dietary changes need to be matched with adjustments to medication. Taking the initially prescribed medication along with a weight loss diet can be dangerous because you can lose control of your sugar levels.

Over the last 15 years in my clinics I have found that the best dietary weight-loss approach to reverse your diabetes is a very low-calorie ketogenic diet (VLCKD). It provides quick and motivating weight loss and is effective in controlling blood sugars.

### How does the VLCKD work?

Of the three macronutrients – carbohydrates, protein and fats – carbohydrates are the preferred choice of energy for our bodies. When you eat carbohydrates, your body either uses them for energy or stores what is not immediately required in the muscles and in the liver, as glycogen. These glycogen stores can be readily accessed when more energy is required. However, if those glycogen stores are full (and they fill up relatively quickly in today's world, when people are constantly eating carbohydrates), the excess carbohydrates will get stored as body fat in adipose tissue, mainly in the middle of the body, around the organs, where it is ready to be turned into energy again. So, to put it simply, you don't have to eat fat to put on fat. Fat is one of the crucial macronutrients, and although eating too much of it can lead to problems, without it we would become ill.

This is a key thing to understand: it's not eating fat that's causing us to get fat, but rather it's the excess carbohydrates that are not being used and that get stored as body fat. That's the problem!

Stored body fat is the most difficult and least preferred source of energy for your body to use. It takes more energy to convert body fat into a reusable form of energy than it takes to get energy out of carbohydrates. Your body will only start to use body fat when it is absolutely necessary. This is why you need to cut down your energy intake, to create a difference between your daily energy needs and your daily energy intake (i.e. calorie deficit). This doesn't mean that you will be low in energy, but that you are not taking in sufficient calories to sustain all your body's requirements, so your body has to start looking for an alternative way to keep you going. Keeping your calorie intake consistently between 800 and 1,000kcal per day and carbohydrate intake to less than 50g per day forces your body to switch to burning body fat. It's like switching from gas to oil!

The VLCKD can seem daunting at first, but when I explain to my patients how it works in practice, they are often surprised by how much there is to eat. Many of them tell me that they eat more on this diet than they have ever eaten before. The diet is so varied

that I very seldom hear patients say that they are getting bored, and if they are, they typically haven't been putting enough effort into cooking the recipes!

When your body uses mainly fat as an energy source, the fat is transformed into ketone bodies. These ketone bodies are the key to your success in sticking to the diet. They suppress your hunger. They give you energy and lift your mood. What's best, though, is that they are a completely normal part of human evolution. If you think about it, we have gone through famine and absence of food without dying. The body keeps going on stored energy and survives.

My practical, tasty and easy-to-follow recipes (see p. 96) make the diet interesting. Most important, you will learn a new way of low-carbohydrate cooking that will help you to stabilise your weight and keep diabetes at bay.

### Why does the VLCKD require supplements?

In order for a VLCKD to be effective and safe, it needs to have the right combination of macronutrients (carbs, protein, fat) and sufficient micronutrients (vitamins and minerals). This is practically impossible to achieve with ordinary food, so the diet is easiest done using a combination of supplements and ordinary foods, mainly vegetables. I use the Eurodiet range as I have found it to be the most comprehensive one available, with a wide variety of choice, providing excellent quality and brand ethos.

It is not the only range of VLCKD supplements on the market and you are welcome to use others; just make sure that they meet the requirements.

Most of the Eurodiet products contain 25% of the dietary reference intake (DRI) of your daily vitamins and minerals and they also contain added fibre. As you will be eating vegetables on the diet, you will get more fibre and nutrients from them.

## What's the difference between low-calorie, low-carbohydrate and ketogenic diets?

It is important to understand that the VLCKD is not just a low-calorie and a low-carbohydrate diet, but also a **ketogenic diet**. While a ketogenic diet is generally referred to as a low-carbohydrate diet, a low-carbohydrate diet is not automatically a ketogenic diet. During a ketogenic diet, you break down your own stored fat, and your body produces these natural 'ketone bodies' that then work as a fuel source.

The type of ketogenic diet I have been using in my clinics is a **high-protein** ketogenic diet, as opposed to a **high-fat** ketogenic diet, which is not specifically designed for weight loss or type 2 diabetes reversal. It is the quick weight loss of a high-protein, low-carbohydrate (around 50g per day) ketogenic diet that appears to be the main driving force in the reversal of type 2 diabetes.

If you were only limiting your calorie and carbohydrate intake (for example during fasting), your body would use all its stores of carbohydrates, proteins and lipids. And once your glycogen stores are depleted, it starts using protein from your muscles as a source of energy. Your muscles are converted to glucose through a process called gluconeogenesis. Instead of losing just body fat, you also lose muscle mass.

Due to the high protein content of the Eurodiet products, your daily protein needs are covered. Not only do they meet your body's daily requirements, they also ensure minimal lean body mass loss and maximum fat loss.

The body can also convert excess protein into glucose, therefore getting energy from it instead of from body fat. This is one of the reasons why eating unlimited amounts of protein is not recommended.

The Eurodiet products also contain significant amounts of omega-3 fatty acids, while keeping the overall fat percentage to less than 30%. I also recommend using some additional oils in cooking. Although good sources of dietary fat are very important, consuming too much can mean that your body gets energy from them instead of from your body fat.

There are many websites and books that explain how to do a ketogenic diet with ordinary foods. This type of food-based diet requires a huge commitment and knowledge of exactly the right types of food you can and cannot eat, as any deviation from these diets can throw you out of ketosis. Our VLCKD is simple and easy to follow and suits someone who doesn't want to start checking everything, and who likes to follow a weekly menu set out for them.

### Why use a high-protein/low-carb diet for treating type 2 diabetes instead of a high-fat/low-carb diet?

In a high-fat, low-carbohydrate ketogenic diet in which calories are not restricted, you get most of your energy from *dietary* fat through ketosis. In a high-protein, low-calorie and low-carbohydrate diet in which the intake of calories and fats is restricted for weight loss purposes, you get the energy from *body* fat through ketosis. In order to reverse type 2 diabetes you need to lose weight and start using body fat as your energy source until you have reversed your condition, or at least achieved improved glycaemic control. Normal sources of protein, such as fish and chicken, have a higher amount of calories than the VLCKD supplements for similar amounts of protein. This is why they are a simple, safe and easy way to get results.

Interestingly, our body, including our brain, can get energy from either glucose (mainly from carbohydrates and sugars) or from ketones (mainly from the breakdown of body fat).

### VLCKD and medication

Most diabetic medications are associated with weight gain (see pp. 56–59) because they work by reducing blood glucose levels: when your blood glucose levels go down, you feel hungry. We eat in response to low blood glucose because that is how our bodies are designed.

The psychological effect of starting medication can also have a detrimental effect on the person's mindset, either by making them feel that now they don't need to do anything about improving their condition themselves, or by making them feel that they have been beaten by their condition and can't do anything about it. I have very rarely seen a patient whose doctor has explained that while they might need medication temporarily (to lower their very high sugar readings at the start of the diagnosis), they should also try to lose weight in order to reduce the visceral fat (hence insulin resistance) as well as their reliance on medication, so that they might be able to come off it. In fact, I think I can count the times I have encountered this on one hand.

On the VLCKD, you can usually stop taking all diabetic *tablet* medication under your doctor's supervision straight away, and seriously reduce your insulin intake (to perhaps only a fifth of what you used to take – but this is highly individual). This gives you a better chance of sticking to the diet because you don't continuously feel the urge to eat. Insulin is a fat-storage hormone:

the more you inject, the less weight you lose. You can't just stop taking your insulin either, so it's up to a qualified and experienced medical professional to find that balance and teach you how to interpret your home glucose readings in order to adjust the dosage accordingly. Witnessing your glucose readings improve without taking diabetic medication is incredibly motivating, with the added benefit that not taking the medication will further increase your weight loss.

When you stop taking the medication, the typical side-effects (see pp. 56–59) start to disappear and you feel much better. No more feeling hungry with your blood sugars going up and down like a rollercoaster. Most people feel less bloated and are clearer in their thinking, instead of having constant 'brain fog'. Chronic tiredness lifts, energy improves dramatically, and aches and pains typically start to lessen, and in some cases disappear completely. Stomach upsets, mood swings and sleep disturbances from waking up to use the bathroom (some medication leads to excess urination) might all be things that you can gladly leave in the past. Many people don't know that the blood sugar rollercoaster can also make sleeping difficult. Balanced blood sugar and ketones can directly improve sleep. In general, when you stop taking the medication, your whole wellbeing improves.

**WARNING: It is dangerous to keep taking certain types of glucose-lowering medication while on the VLCKD. Your glucose levels may drop too low and result in a hypo.**

When you start the VLCKD, your doctor can typically stop all your diabetic *tablet* medications immediately and either reduce or stop your insulin intake. The blood sugar medication was initially used to help lower your blood sugars while you were eating the way you used to. On the new regime of VLCKD, the same level of medications could bring your blood sugars dangerously low because the blood sugars get lower naturally during the diet. Therefore, you should discuss coming off your medication with your doctor before starting the diet and explain that you are going on a low-carbohydrate diet. Some doctors might not necessarily be familiar with the diet and perhaps might not immediately be in favour of you doing it – many doctors lack experience of using the diet to improve type 2 diabetes. You could show them this book to help them understand that you can't take medication while you are on this diet. It is important that once you start the diet, you stick to it, as it is impossible for your doctor to adjust and lower your medication if you are not sticking to the plan and keeping your blood sugars under control.

Reducing or stopping medication gives you a better chance of sticking to the diet because you don't continuously feel the urge to eat.

Ideally, your doctor will take your bloods (fasting glucose, HbA1c and others, depending on your medical situation) before you start on the diet and again in the following weeks (2–4 weeks, depending on your doctor's decision and the level of support he/she considers you need and is able to give you). The aim of repeating the bloods within a short period of time is to ensure that your glucose control improves, or at least stays the same (as at the beginning of the diet) with reduced or no medication. This proves that the diet is working.

Once you start coming off the VLCKD and reintroduce carbohydrates (ideally doing this slowly, and following the Phase 3 plan for some time), your doctor should take the HbA1c again, and repeat this when you have been off the VLCKD for 3–4 weeks, and again three months after you have come off the VLCKD. You have only officially managed to reverse type 2 diabetes when you can tolerate carbohydrates without your fasting sugars and HbA1c going above normal levels. It should be noted that while some people can return to eating some carbohydrates throughout the day, others may need to be more mindful and keep the portions small. Regardless, the quality and quantity of your choices, along with factors such as physical activity, make a big difference.

Depending on how much weight (visceral fat) you have lost, your reduced insulin resistance and how much insulin production was left in your pancreas at the end of the diet, your doctor will be able to review your glucose-lowering medication requirements. As you saw in the Case Studies section, some people, especially those who embarked on the weight loss diet at the very beginning of their diabetes diagnoses, e.g. James Kelly (p. 19), were able to stay off the medication completely, even when they reintroduced more carbo-hydrates into their daily diet. On the other hand, Pat Mulcahy and Brendan Coyne still required a small amount of daily oral glucose-lowering medication when they moved to a maintenance diet.

# What to Expect

My average patient needs to lose 3 stone (19kg) to reverse their type 2 diabetes.

Everyone's medical history and metabolism are different, so I can't promise how many pounds/kilograms someone might lose in a set timeframe. However, from experience we can see that on the VLCKD, people typically tend to lose 10% of their starting weight in 6–8 weeks, and men usually lose it faster than women. This is only if the person sticks strictly to the diet, of course.

There are many reasons why people sometimes deviate from the diet: not having time to prepare meals in advance, holidays, social arrangements, travelling for work, sick children or other domestic challenges, and so on. However, with some support and tips, it should be possible to stick to the diet even in those situations. You just need to realise that all of those things do influence the time it takes to reach your first 10% goal.

There are no set rules as to how long people stay on the VLCKD or the various phases of the diet; this is driven by many individual factors. We have seen many patients – especially if they have a lot of weight to lose – stay on Phase 1 of the diet for several months, while others might decide to switch to Phase 2 after only a couple of weeks. Usually, when they switch phases, people accept a slowing of weight loss as well.

Once people start feeling some benefits, it is easier to be motivated to stick to the diet. Usually with weight loss comes extra energy, more mobility, less bloating and less joint pain, among other things, which are extra motivating factors.

The most inspiring aspect of the diet, however, can be when the person sees for themselves that their blood sugar readings (glucose and HbA1c) are the same or lower without medication. It is then that people fully realise that weight loss, diet and lifestyle have a huge impact on overall glucose control. Most people feel a sense of empowerment and see that, with their new diet and lifestyle, they can change their health, reverse their diabetes and improve their health destiny.

## What if weight loss is not as fast as expected?

Weight loss can seem incredibly daunting, but it's actually quite simple: the bigger the difference between the calories your body needs and the calorie intake, the bigger the weight loss. The lower the carbohydrate intake, the faster the weight loss. So if you stick to the plan, you *will* lose weight.

Keep in mind, too, that you will get lighter all the time, so you cannot expect the same weekly weight loss when you have already lost a lot! Instead, you should count your weight loss as a percentage of your starting weight, to make sure you're on the right track.

If you think you're doing everything right and sticking to the plan *every day*, and the weight loss is not fast enough, look at the following possible issues.

## Are you getting too many calories?
- Cut back on the 'extra luxury items', such as coconut milk in curry or cheese in soup or bread.
- Choose lower-calorie Eurodiet products.
- Measure your daily oil intake (1–2 tbsp per day).
- Measure your portion of protein (from Phase 2 onwards).

## Are you getting too many carbohydrates?
- Choose vegetables from List 1 only (p. 97).
- Choose lower-carbohydrate Eurodiet products.
- Keep your vegetable intake under 800g a day.
- Substitute some of the vegetables with Konjac spaghetti or rice.

## Are you getting 'hidden sugars' from somewhere else?
- Check that your soy sauce contains no sugar – look at in the ingredients list.
- Cut back or leave out any seasoning that may be a culprit (such as balsamic vinegar).
- Limit milk in tea or coffee.

## Are you drinking too many caffeinated drinks or having some alcohol?
- Keep your caffeine intake to a minimum (1–2 hot caffeinated drinks a day).
- Avoid diet drinks if you think this is having an impact.
- Alcohol has calories, even if it's low in sugar.

## Are you exercising too much or being extremely sedentary?
- Strenuous exercise is not recommended during the VLCKD.
- You could try walking 30 minutes a day.

## Other possible reasons for slower than expected weight loss:
- **Medication** can impact your body's ability to lose weight: some possible culprits are beta blockers, diabetic drugs, anti-depressants and anti-psychotic drugs, hormones (oestrogen), drugs to treat arthritis, pain medications, steroids, Tamoxifen.
- **Medical issues** such as hypothyroidism, or an inadequate dose of medication used to treat this condition.
- **Menstrual cycle:** weekly weight loss on the week of a period is often less than expected.
- **Inadequate sleep** may lead you to take in more calories without noticing and to choose higher-calorie and higher-carbo-hydrate foods; your hormones will be out of balance, which could trigger your body to eat more and to store fat.
- **Chronic stress:** the hormone cortisol is elevated with chronic stress, and this can

both influence your behaviour around food and also hormonally influence your body's ability to lose weight.

**Tips for dealing with constipation**
Constipation can happen at any time, to anyone, when their routine changes. The most likely changes in routine that result in constipation are dietary changes, travel and changes in activity patterns.

Medication and changes in medication can also cause constipation, and often people don't realise this. Painkillers, antacids, anti-depressants and even some blood pressure medications can make you constipated. Iron and calcium supplements may also be a problem. If you think your medications or supplements are causing a problem, talk to your doctor.

Some medical conditions are associated with constipation. Hypothyroidism (underactive thyroid) is perhaps the most common, and this should be investigated.

If constipation starts to trouble you when you start your new diet, follow this guide to eliminate possible causes and find relief with some simple solutions.

**Check your fibre intake** (aim for minimum of 25g fibre/day)
- Are you making soup and having it daily?
- Are you including sufficient high-fibre vegetables at dinnertime?
- If you are eating salads, are you adding high-fibre vegetables to them, such as peppers, broccoli, cabbage, fennel, asparagus, etc.?
- Have you increased your fibre intake but not your water intake at the same time?

**Check your fluid intake**
- Are you drinking the recommended 2 litres of water daily?
- Have you suddenly stopped drinking coffee, or increased your coffee or tea consumption? Too much of either can slow things down, and some people find that coffee, in particular, is like a gentle laxative.
- Are you drinking too much water at mealtimes or after meals? This can slow down proper digestion.

**Physical activity**
- Are you very sedentary? A sedentary lifestyle increases the chances of constipation.
- Movement and exercise – even going for a walk – may help stimulate peristalsis (the natural muscle contractions of the gut).

**Good dietary fats**
- Are you getting the recommended 1–2 tbsp of good oils daily?

**Some additional tips that may help**
- Try 1 tbsp flaxseed or 1–2 tsp psyllium husks daily.
- Try stewed rhubarb (sweetened with Xylitol or Stevia).
- Avoid red meat and choose oily fish (from Phase 2 onwards).

- Choose (Eurodiet) products with higher fibre content.

**If the above dietary changes do not provide relief, also consider:**
- Gentle laxative tea
- Magnesium citrate supplement
- Probiotics
- Digestive aids.

**And don't forget the basics**
- Give yourself time to visit the bathroom, especially in the morning.
- Chew your food well and avoid eating on the go.

# The Plan

The are four phases to the plan:

- Phase 1 and Phase 2 are the ketogenic part of the diet. This means that your body starts using its own fat stores for energy. You will eat less than 50g carbohydrates a day.
- Phase 3 is the non-ketogenic stage of the diet. Carbohydrates exceed 50g but you are still in an energy deficit and losing weight. You can also start exercising on this phase.
- The Maintenance Phase follows, in which you go back to eating a balanced healthy diet without the need for Eurodiet supplements.

The main difference between Phase 1 and Phase 2 is that on Phase 2, the protein for your main meal comes from an ordinary source and not a Eurodiet supplement. This makes it slightly higher in calories and requires a bit more organising and control.

Vegetables form the basis of my VLCKD Plan and the Eurodiet supplements are there to provide the protein, vitamins, minerals and additional fibre without the extra calories and carbohydrates. I typically recommend 700–800g (approx. 1.5lb) of vegetables every day. To make sure you reach your recommended daily fibre intake, choose vegetables that grow overground.

On p. 97 there are two lists of vegetables. List 1 vegetables contain less carbohydrates, so on Phases 1 and 2, two-thirds of your vegetable intake should come from List 1 and one-third from List 2. On Phase 3 onwards you can start including some root vegetables.

You can start either on Phase 1 or Phase 2 but typically people start on Phase 1 as the weight loss is quicker.

While it is not necessary or realistic to leave out carbohydrates for the rest of your life, it is safe to cut the amount right down for a short period of time in order to lose weight.

However, you cannot leave out protein, and it tends to be safer to eat a little more protein than too little protein. But remember, because you are diabetic you need to keep your carbohydrate intake under control. The way I explain it is that you have an 'intolerance' to carbohydrates, so too much is clearly not good for you!

**Drinks**

Drink about 2–2.5 litres (4–5 pints) of water a day. I recommend that you cut down on tea, coffee and diet drinks without any radical changes at first. I suggest 2–3 cups a day at most. If you like your tea or coffee with sugar, use a sweetener like Xylitol or Stevia, and ideally do not add milk. Milk contains lactose (milk sugar), and this could negatively affect ketosis.

I find sparkling water to be particularly refreshing with a slice of lemon.

**Eurodiet supplements**

I prefer this range as it has a good variety and I have come to trust the brand. There are over 90 products, with gluten-free and vegetarian options, and both savoury and sweet options. While they are formulated to look and taste as close to ordinary food as possible, they have a completely different nutritional composition. Below are some examples of the differences between the nutrient content of ordinary food and the Eurodiet equivalent.

You can see from the table that the Eurodiet supplements have a lower carbohydrate content and a higher protein content than ordinary food. They are enriched with the vitamins and minerals you won't get from food when you cut out entire food groups, such as fruit, grains and dairy.

In the phase sample plans, be aware that a Eurodiet 'snack' is usually only half a large bar or a few biscuits from a pack of six.

| Example (per 100g) | kcal | Carbs | Protein | Fibre |
|---|---|---|---|---|
| Ordinary porridge | 371 | 64 | 11 | 8 |
| Eurodiet porridge | 376 | 25 | 50 | 7 |
| Brown bread | 203 | 44 | 8 | 4 |
| Eurodiet bread | 248 | 4 | 30 | 13 |
| Brown pasta | 321 | 60 | 14 | 8 |
| Eurodiet pasta | 350 | 20 | 60 | 3.5 |
| Chocolate biscuits | 497 | 61 | 7 | 4 |
| Eurodiet biscuits | 427 | 24 | 31 | 14 |

# Phase 1

Phase 1 is a very low-carbohydrate ketogenic diet (VLCKD). On this phase you should go into ketosis within three or four days. Your diabetic medication will need to be reduced or stopped under medical supervision.

The Phase 1 daily formula is made up as follows:

- 700–800g (1.5–1.7lb) of vegetables (see p. 97 for a list).
- 4–5 Eurodiet products a day.
- Take one to two electrolyte supplements (Laktolight; see p. 77) to ensure optimal balance of electrolytes.
- You need to add some salt to your food because sodium is an important electrolyte.
- 1–2 tbsp of good-quality oils, e.g. olive oil.
- At least 1.5–2 litres of water (light herbal teas can be counted towards this total).

Take a look at the sample menu plan for Phase 1 (see p. 76) to get an understanding of the principles of the plan. As long as you follow the recommended principles and formula, you can freely choose between the products and vegetables. Most people batch-cook and freeze one or two soups and some of the vegetable dishes at the weekend and take them out as needed. It is also perfectly fine to use frozen vegetables!

Go through the sample plan and decide what suits you best. If you're in a rush in the morning and don't typically have a big **breakfast**, you might like to make the Eurodiet tropical smoothie the night before and just grab it from the fridge on your way out. If you have time for something more substantial, try the Eurodiet omelette with some vegetables. Some people just have the Eurodiet porridge for breakfast, and that's okay; you don't necessarily need variety if it makes life complicated.

I would always recommend a good serving of vegetables for **lunch**, and the easiest way to ensure that you have something substantial is to batch-cook soups at the weekend. A typical Eurodiet product to have with soup for lunch is the organic Eurodiet bread or crackers with some light cheese. If you like salads, you need to include 300–400g of crunchy vegetables, such as broccoli, celery and peppers, as well as some leaves to get enough fibre. You can follow the recipes in this book (see p. 95) or make up your own soups and salads using the allowed lists of vegetables (see p. 97).

At **snack times** you can have a portion of a sweet snack, such as some of the Eurodiet biscuits or chocolate squares, with a hot or cold drink. If you prefer a savoury snack, you could try the chilli nuts, or dip the Eurodiet breadsticks into my Mediterranean dip (see p. 213). There are so many flavours, textures and varieties to choose from that it's very difficult to get bored! At any time, you can also have more vegetables in any shape or form from the allowed list (see p. 97).

**Dinner** can take several forms. It could include the Eurodiet pasta or Eurodiet burger with Moroccan-spiced vegetables (see p. 210). Some people prefer to make a vegetable curry (see p. 214) with the Konjac zero-carbohydrate noodles, and then have one of the Eurodiet desserts or hot drinks for the protein.

## Phase 1: Sample Plan

|  | Day 1 | Day 2 | Day 3 |
|---|---|---|---|
| **Breakfast** | Eurodiet Porridge made with Laktolight, served with stewed rhubarb (p. 106) | Eurodiet Frittata (p. 153) | Eurodiet crêpe made with Laktolight and a sprinkle of cinnamon |
| **Snack** | 2 Eurodiet raspberry biscuits | Eurodiet chocolate muffin | ½ bag of Eurodiet jellies |
| **Lunch** | Creamy Veg Soup (p. 138) with Eurodiet bread (p. 120), a scraping of soft cheese and cucumber slices | Creamy Mushroom Soup (p. 142) with 5 Eurodiet crispy toasts and 1 portion of light Laughing Cow cheese | Eurodiet Pasta Salad served with pesto (p. 122) |
| **Snack** | Eurodiet coconut mini bar | 2 Eurodiet raspberry biscuits | ½ bag of Eurodiet jellies |
| **Dinner** | Eurodiet pasta with Tomato and Vegetable Sauce (p. 209) | Eurodiet pizza (p. 154) | Stir-fry with Turmeric and Chilli (p. 215) |
| **Snack** | 2 Eurodiet raspberry biscuits | Eurodiet chocolate pot | Eurodiet vanilla rice pudding |

## Laktolight

You should consume two Laktolight sachets each day during Phase 1 and Phase 2, and ideally one a day during Phase 3 of the VLCKD. Laktolight is a low-calorie, low-sugar, calcium- and potassium-enriched milk powder that makes products bulkier and more pleasant. It is very important to use it during the fast weight loss part because it contains minerals that you might otherwise be too low on. Side-effects of not using Laktolight can include leg cramps, headaches and general tiredness.

Most Eurodiet products are easy to prepare with Laktolight. You can also make the products with water, and have the Laktolight as a drink or as a milk substitute in tea and coffee. Some people add Laktolight to their heated soup at lunchtime.

If you have any of the following rare conditions, or are taking medications or supplements, please advise your healthcare professional.

- Hypersensitivity to potassium
- Kidney failure
- Addison's disease
- Hyperkalemia
- Any conditions associated with hypercalcaemia and hypercalciuria
- If you are taking potassium-saving diuretics.

# Phase 2

While you are still on a VLCKD and remain in ketosis, in this phase you replace one of the main meal Eurodiet protein elements with an ordinary source of protein, e.g. 200g white fish, 150g meat (see the table on p. 80 for a full list).

This phase gives more flexibility for those who travel or eat out a lot as it allows one main meal with ordinary protein, which is easy to get at a restaurant. It also suits a group meal situation – you can still join in the meal but just avoid the carbohydrate portion.

As you are still in ketosis, you should see no increase in your home sugar readings. They should actually be improving all the time! There are more calories in the ordinary source of protein, and possibly in the oil it's cooked in, so you can expect the rate of weight loss to slow down slightly.

The Phase 2 daily formula is as follows:

- 700g–800g (1.5–1.7lb) of vegetables (two-thirds from List 1, one-third from List 2).
- 1 portion of protein for your main meal.
- 3–4 Eurodiet supplements per day.
- 1–2 Laktolight to ensure electrolyte balance.
- Add salt to your food.
- 1–2 tbsp of good-quality oils (e.g. olive oil).
- At least 2 litres (4–5pints) of water.

You can also start the VLCKD from Phase 2. Although you may get a less significant weight loss boost right from the start, your sugar readings are still likely to start reducing. Some people find Phase 1 too difficult because they feel they need a piece of meat, chicken or fish to be satisfied. You can always try Phase 1 for just few days, and see if you like it. If you don't, it doesn't mean that you have failed. Just continue on Phase 2 instead.

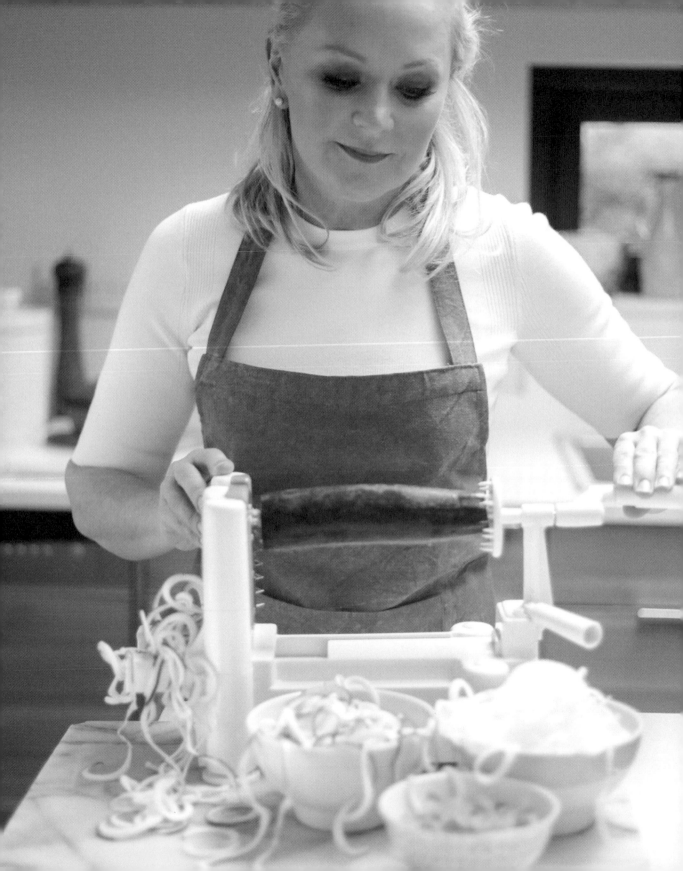

| Protein | Portion |
|---|---|
| Red meat (e.g. beef), pork, lamb, game (e.g. venison), organ meats (e.g. liver) | 120g/4oz |
| Oily fish (salmon, tuna, trout, mackerel, sardines, herring, anchovies) | 120g/4oz |
| Tinned oily fish (in brine or water only, drained weight) | 120g/4oz |
| Poultry (chicken, turkey, duck) | 150g/5oz |
| White fish (all varieties, e.g. cod, haddock, hake, sea bass, monkfish) | 200g/7oz |
| Tinned white fish or seafood (in brine or water only, drained weight) | 200g/7oz |
| Eggs | 2 large |
| Tofu* with high soybean content (over 30%) | 150g/5oz |
| Quorn chicken or mince* | 120g/4oz |
| Cheeses* | see p. 99 for portions |

*Please note that tofu, Quorn products and cheese contain some carbohydrates.*

## Phase 2 sample meal plan

| | Day 1 | Day 2 | Day 3 |
|---|---|---|---|
| **Breakfast** | Eurodiet Omelette made with Laktolight and 200g of wilted spinach (p. 102) | Eurodiet tropical smoothie made with Laktolight (p. 114) | Eurodiet Strawberry Chia Pudding (p. 109) |
| **Snack** | ½ Eurodiet hazelnut caramel bar | 2 Eurodiet raspberry biscuits | ½ bag Eurodiet jellies |
| **Lunch** | Asparagus and Blue Cheese Soup (p. 134) with Eurodiet croûtons | Eurodiet Egg Fried Rice (p. 150) | Cauliflower and Celery Soup with Spices (p. 135), and 3 slices Eurodiet toast |
| **Snack** | ½ Eurodiet hazelnut caramel bar | 2 Eurodiet raspberry biscuits | ½ bag Eurodiet jellies |
| **Dinner** | Lamb and Feta Burgers (p. 168) with Cauliflower Rice (p. 196) and rocket salad | Spicy Chicken and Vegetable Casserole (p. 158) | Aubergine Pizzas (p. 206) with roasted vegetables |
| **Snack** | Eurodiet chocolate muffin | 2 Eurodiet raspberry biscuits | Ready-made sugar-free jelly |

# Phase 3

Depending on your final weight loss goal and current home blood glucose readings, you may be able to introduce ordinary foods much sooner than you had expected. You are still creating an energy deficit in this plan as your calorie intake is between 1,000 and 1,200 kcal per day, so most people will still lose some weight.

In Phase 3 you replace one more Eurodiet product with a portion of carbohydrates and some ordinary protein, and introduce a portion of fruit.

The daily Phase 3 formula is as follows:

- 500–600g (1.1–1.3lb) vegetables from Lists 1 and 2 (see p. 97); but you can now occasionally have onion, carrots, peas, butternut squash, parsnip, beetroot, etc.
- Two Eurodiet products, typically one 'meal'-type (such as the porridge, bread or omelette) and one 'snack'-type (such as a packet of biscuits or one large bar).
- One Laktolight supplement.
- One large portion of protein for your main meal (already introduced in Phase 2).
- Another, smaller portion of protein (half of the value of Phase 2 main meal (see p. 80)
- A portion of fruit (see p. 84).
- A portion of carbohydrates (see p. 84).
- Add salt to taste.
- 1–2 tbsp of good-quality oils and fats.
- Aim for 1.5–2 litres (3–4 pints) of water every day.

Replacing one Eurodiet supplement with carbohydrates and ordinary protein can be done at any meal, but ideally you should do it at either breakfast or lunch as you are more active during the day. You may want to start having some porridge (carbohydrates) with milk (protein), and then have the Eurodiet organic bread at lunchtime with your soup. Or you could have some real bread (carbohydrates) with ham (protein) at lunchtime with soup, and have Eurodiet porridge for breakfast. Although most people like my carbohydrate substitutes at dinner, such as Pilau Cauliflower Rice (p. 201) or Turnip Chips with Cajun Seasoning (p. 202), you could choose to have a portion of potato, rice or pasta at dinnertime instead, with a source of protein.

This is when it gets a little more complicated, but if you have made it this far, I'm sure you can get to grips with this new phase. The serving sizes for protein at your main meal time in Phase 3 are the same as in Phase 2 (see p. 80). The carbohydrate choices are (almost!) endless, as you will see on p. 84.

## Phase 3 sample meal plan

|  | Day 1 | Day 2 | Day 3 |
|---|---|---|---|
| **Breakfast** | 40g oats made into porridge with 200ml milk | Eurodiet Porridge made with Laktolight | Tropical Breakfast Smoothie (p. 114) |
| **Snack** | Apple | Eurodiet chocolate crispy bar | Eurodiet muffin dip |
| **Lunch** | Chorizo and Cauliflower Soup (p. 137) with Eurodiet bread, light cheese and peppers | Finn Crisp Rolls with Cream Cheese (p. 125) and Raw Power Salad (p. 119) | Chicken Fajitas (p. 192) |
| **Snack** | 2 Eurodiet chocolate biscuits | 2 plums | 2 Eurodiet chocolate biscuits |
| **Dinner** | Turkey and Horseradish Burgers (p. 175) | Yuk Sung with Spicy Cabbage (p. 159) | Jambalaya (p. 172) |
| **Snack** | Crudités with Mediterranean dip (p. 213) | ½ bag Eurodiet sweet chilli crisps | ½ bag Eurodiet sweet chilli crisps |

## Carbohydrate suggestions for breakfast

Here are some ideas for breakfast carbohydrates, which should be around 150kcal per serving and typical proteins to serve with them (approximately 100kcal per serving).

- 40g grain-based unsweetened cereals, such as oats, buckwheat, barley, cereal mixes, muesli or 2 pieces of low-sugar breakfast 'biscuits' with 150–200ml milk, natural yogurt or egg.
- 1–2 pieces of wholemeal bread or bagel with 60g smoked salmon, egg, 2 slices cold meats or cheese.

## Carbohydrate suggestions for lunch

For lunch, you should have approximately 150kcal per serving from carbohydrates. Typical proteins to serve with them should be approximately 100kcal per serving. For example:

- 2–4 wholemeal crackers, or
- wholemeal pitta pocket or wrap, or
- 1–2 pieces of wholemeal bread, or
- 100g cooked quinoa, brown rice or pasta.

## Served with:

- 60–80g cooked chicken, meat or oily fish, or
- 100g cooked seafood or white fish, or
- 2–3 slices of cold lean deli meats
- 1 egg
- ½ portion of any cheese (see p. 99 for list)
- ½ portion of any Phase 2 dinner portions

- 100g cooked legumes (chickpeas, lentils, butterbeans, etc., but note that these also contain carbohydrates)

## Carbohydrate suggestions for dinner

For dinner, the calories from carbohydrates should not exceed 170kcal per serving. For example:

- 1 medium potato or sweet potato
- 50g (uncooked weight) brown rice, wholemeal pasta, noodles or quinoa
- wholemeal wrap or pitta pocket
- 150g cooked legumes

## Fruit portions

On Phase 3 you can have fruit once a day, but you should keep the portion to about 50–70kcal. This would typically be:

- 1 medium (palm-sized) fruit, such as apple, orange, pear, kiwi
- 1–2 smaller fruits, such as plum, nectarine, apricot, peach
- 100–150g of any berries or currants.

## Glucose control when introducing more carbohydrates

It is important to note that I always repeat the HbA1c blood test before my patients start Phase 3. I do it again after a few weeks, while the patient monitors home glucose readings at the same time. This enables me to monitor the patient's glucose control and make a judgement on whether or not they can tolerate carbohydrates, whether they have reversed their diabetes, or if I need to start them on some oral hypoglycaemic medication. Should this happen, it is highly unlikely that you would need to go back to the same amount of medication, especially if you are willing to embrace a lower-than-usual carbohydrate lifestyle along with physical exercise.

Ideally, you need to start introducing the new foods slowly. This will help you to control your behaviour and hunger. The ketogenic Phases 1 and 2 will have suppressed your hunger, and sometimes people notice normal hunger (before mealtimes) when starting Phase 3. Increased carbohydrates may increase your blood sugar readings and sometimes make you crave carbohydrates, but this really depends on the person. Introducing a wider variety of ordinary foods requires more discipline: with more 'freedom' in your diet, you could be more tempted to go off the plan.

There is no set time when people are ready to switch to Phase 3, but ideally your fasting glucose and HbA1c should have come down to non-diabetic levels. However, this does not necessarily mean that you can only switch to Phase 3 once your weight has come down. It is important to understand that in Phase 3 you are going to introduce carbohydrates and this means losing the benefits of ketosis, especially the hunger suppression.

As we are introducing more carbohydrates in this phase, it is also important to start exercising regularly. We recommend a minimum of 30 minutes of exercise daily. It's best to find something that you enjoy and can stick to.

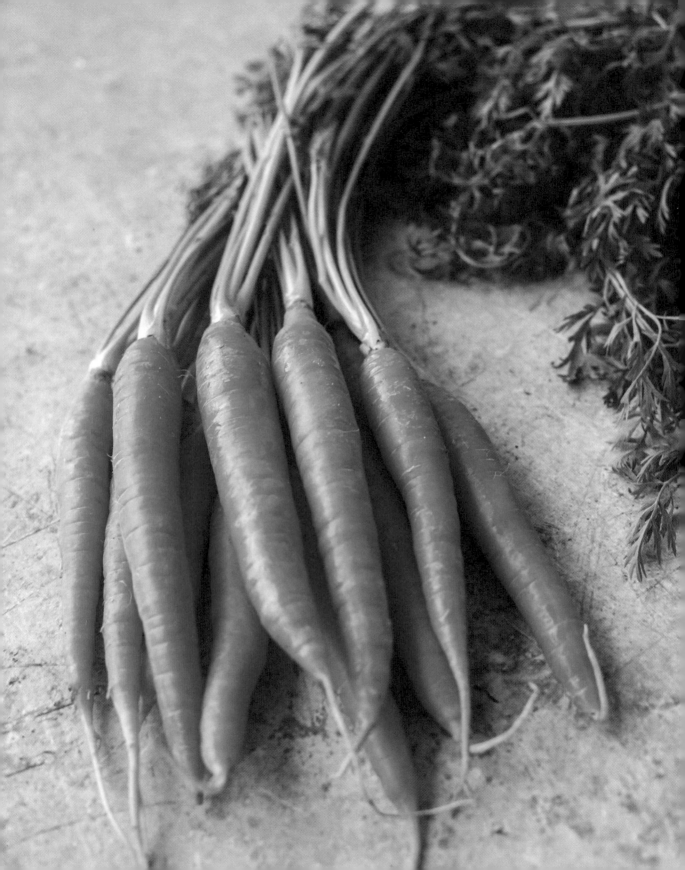

# Maintenance

Congratulations! You have reversed your type 2 diabetes, or at least significantly improved your glucose control by losing sufficient weight to achieve this. You should now have stopped all your diabetic medication or at least significantly reduced it. After Phase 3 you can start moving on to the maintenance plan without the help of the Eurodiet supplements. It is very important on the maintenance plan to start looking at the calorie, carbohydrate, protein and sugar content of foods to ensure that you do not start gaining weight and lose your improved glucose control.

When people finish 'dieting', they often feel as if they have just been released from a dieting prison and they can now go wild and eat anything they want. This is not the right approach. You need to actively work on continually reminding yourself of your incredible achievement. Of course you had to avoid certain foods and treats in the first three phases, but now you must understand that not all calories are equal and some are absorbed more rapidly than others. Once you have consumed the calories, they are in your body. While some people seem to be able to revert to eating carbohydrates at each meal, others may find that their weight and their glucose readings go up. This is why it is crucial to monitor your progress and adjust what, how much and when you're eating.

Instead of thinking about how many calories you can afford to have each day, you may find it easier to imagine that the calories are like money. Let's say you wake up each morning with €2,000 in your wallet and this is the maximum amount of money you have to spend for the whole day. If you want to spend it wisely and not end up in debt – or in calorie terms, gain weight – you need to plan and track how you are spending it.

You could choose to spend €300 on breakfast and have €1,700 for the rest of the day. Likewise, if you spend €1,400 first thing on a full Irish breakfast, you would definitely struggle to spend only €600 for the rest of the day!

When trying to maintain weight, it is crucial that you are aware of how you distribute these units of energy throughout the day. It is amazing how quickly they can add up, especially when certain products give the impression of being healthy or a better choice by labelling such as 'reduced fat', 'high protein', 'no added sugar', 'lower calorie', 'gluten-free' and so on.

Here's an example of how quickly the calories can clock up. A breakfast consisting of one slice of wholemeal bread, poached egg, a scrape of butter and a cup of tea with milk would be approximately 250kcals. If you had a nice bowl of homemade soup with two wholemeal crackers and a tin of sardines for lunch, this would be approximately 400kcals. Then a simple dinner consisting of a boiled chicken fillet, brown basmati rice, steamed vegetables and a side salad with a drizzle of olive oil would most likely add up to around 750kcals. If you snacked on two regular pieces of fruit and a few nuts with yoghurt, your daily total spend would already be around 1,800kcal.

Although this example sounds like something aimed at weight loss, the calorie intake is already over 1,600kcals, which is the Food Safety Authority of Ireland's (FSAI) daily recommendation for an average older sedentary female; men can typically afford around 200kcal more. Yet the food industry labels food products based on a guideline daily amount (GDA) of 2,000kcal, which is really based on someone who is of an average height and moderately active. This level of daily calorie consumption would be too much for the majority of people.

You can see how misleading GDAs can be and how these guidelines can easily make you feel that you are doing quite well. If, for example, you pick up a takeaway cappuccino at the petrol station and grab a typical chocolate bar to go with it, you might glance at the bar's calorie content but forget about the calories in the cappuccino. Similarly, you might get a low-calorie, healthy salad from one of the many new salad bars that include a calorie count on the menu, but then add some extras, such as boiled egg, toasted seeds and avocado. Although these are so-called 'good calories', they will add a couple of hundred calories to your lunch.

Most of us underestimate the amount of calories we take in every day. Believe me, I know all about it. My personal calorie requirement on a day when I am not very physically active is most likely below 1,600kcal, which can be difficult not to go over, especially when my weakness is chocolate!

But instead of feeling sorry for ourselves, we need to be actively involved in maintaining our weight. There's no point comparing yourself to anyone else; we each have a unique requirement that is based on factors from our past and present life. In fact, there are many factors that you have to consider before estimating your daily calorie requirements, such as age, gender, height, weight, level of activity, medication, illnesses and past diets.

As a general rule of thumb, in order to maintain your current weight there must be an energy balance. In other words, the amount of calories you consume should match the amount of calories you expend throughout the day. I use Tanita bioimpedance scales in my clinics to assess each patient's personal daily calorie requirement. Although no method can be 100% reliable, this machine is able to assess your body composition, taking into account some of the above factors, as well as your lean body tissue and fat tissue. In a print-out report it gives your body fat percentage, fat mass, muscle mass, water weight, bone mass, metabolic age, visceral fat rating, body mass index (BMI), your ideal body weight with recommended body fat percentage and your current basal metabolic rate (BMR). BMR is the number of calories your body needs to keep it functioning at rest. Based on this, we are able to create a suitable maintenance diet plan for each person.

BMR varies incredibly from person to person. For example, a 22-year-old man measuring 90kg (14st) and 180cm (approx. 5ft 9in) could have a BMR of 2,050kcal. His daily calorie requirements would increase with exercise, meaning we could roughly calculate that he can multiply his BMR by 1.4 on the days that he is active, giving him a lot more calories to spend! On the other hand, a 70-year-old man who weighs the same but is only 165cm (5ft 4in) would have a BMR of approximately 1,600kcal.

It can actually take some trial and error, even for us professionals, to figure out a maintenance plan with a sufficient amount of calories that will also stop you from losing more weight. A great example of this is a lady in her seventies with type 2 diabetes who came to the clinic not so long ago. On our plan, she lost a perfect amount of weight and reversed her type 2 diabetes. With this success, and considering her age, gender and weight, we thought she could only eat maybe 1,400–1,600kcal per day in order to maintain her weight. However, she was still losing some weight when she started her maintenance plan, which meant that we had to actively keep adding more good calories. Lucky her!

Your BMR decreases with weight loss as the body needs fewer calories to maintain a smaller person, but it typically drops more dramatically when people just cut back on calories in order to lose weight, without taking much notice of where these calories come from. We are able to monitor this progress and advise our patients accordingly. This is why it is vital for your future maintenance to know what is happening during weight loss: are you losing fat or are you losing muscle?

A pound of muscle and a pound of fat are obviously the same weight, but in reality they have different requirements for calories. It is more beneficial to have a higher percentage of muscle than fat. Consequently, I focus on helping you lower your fat mass during your weight loss while maintaining, or even *increasing*, your muscle mass. This is where the emphasis on protein is important and the reason why the VLCKD is a valuable tool: your body sees the stored fat as the main source of fuel and uses it to meet the daily energy requirement created by the deficit. Of course, the Eurodiet supplements, and vegetables, contain calories, but they are also making sure that you meet your daily protein, fibre and micronutrient requirements while keeping fats and carbohydrates at the minimum requirement levels.

Many factors have an effect on how energy is released from your food and also how food is digested. However, you can do very little about these factors. You may have heard of the glycaemic index (GI). It was invented in 1981 by David Jenkins, a professor of nutrition at the University of Toronto, to help people with diabetes. It is a tool we use to establish how quickly certain foods affect your blood glucose readings.

For example, if you had white rice, which has a higher GI than brown rice, with a food that contains protein *and* fat (e.g. salmon), and served it with vegetables containing fibre, you would feel fuller than you would if you ate the same amount of calories from rice alone, and your postprandial (after a meal) blood sugars would be more stable.

Low-GI carbohydrates – like wholemeal bread instead of white bread – are much more beneficial than high-GI carbohydrates not only because they have a higher nutrient content, but also because their glucose is released and metabolised at a much slower rate than glucose from high-GI carbs. The glucose from high-GI carbs is released much faster and is used by the body faster, creating a spike in blood sugar levels and temporary hunger satisfaction. When these blood sugar levels fall, which happens a lot more quickly than when you eat low-GI foods, hunger and cravings come back and you start looking for the next quick hit, leading to overeating throughout the day.

Low and high GI can be complicated and confusing as it is very seldom that you eat only one type of food. I would rather you focus on the following principles during your weight maintenance:

- Have some protein at each meal, including at snack time.
- Choose a carbohydrate source that contains a good quantity of fibre.
- Include additional fibre from vegetables.
- Make sure the bulk of your meals comes from low-carbohydrate vegetables.
- Enjoy some good fats.

I want to encourage you to plan your meals with all this in mind. I cannot give you exact portions as I don't know how many calories you need to maintain your weight, or if you have any intolerances or beliefs that limit your food choices. But if you were eating an average, broad diet, like the example on pp. 87–88 (where I show how calories clock up), you would get some protein and fat from your egg at breakfast, and if you choose a good-quality, wholemeal, high-fibre bread to eat with the egg, and added some sliced vegetables and salad leaves, you would have addressed all the main principles for that meal.

Activity levels before and after you eat also play a part, both in your glucose readings and in weight management. Your glycogen stores are less full after an overnight fast, so, for example, if you eat a regular portion of foods containing carbohydrates in the morning, you are less likely to store any excess carbohydrate breakdown product (glucose) as fat because it will typically just 'fill' those glycogen stores instead. Also keep in mind that if you have reduced your activity levels, you will most likely need to reduce your daily calorie intake. For example, if you used to walk 20 minutes a day to and from work but because you have changed your job you are now driving, you have reduced your weekly activity levels by over three hours. Likewise, if you suffer an injury and are required to stay completely sedentary, your calorie requirement would almost equate to your basic BMR.

People may think that when an exercise machine, such as a treadmill or rowing machine, tells them they have burned 300 calories, it is accurate information. It is not. It's just a very rough estimate and should be taken with a pinch of salt. Nearly all exercise machines don't take account of important factors such as your weight, age and fitness level, which is a huge factor. For example, a 90kg man with a low fitness level versus a 75kg man with a high fitness level would burn a totally different amount of calories doing the same exercise for 30 minutes.

Sleep is also a factor we tend to underestimate when it comes to managing our weight (see Sleep Apnoea on p. 43). When you sleep, your body and mind are at rest and have time to recharge. On average, most people require between six and eight hours of good-quality sleep every night. Any less than this, or having poor-quality sleep, makes a significant difference to how you feel physically and emotionally, and impacts your behaviour towards food the next day. The production of several hormones becomes disrupted and because of this your body's functioning changes,

making you act and feel differently from normal. For example, leptin (a hormone that signals satiety) levels go down, while levels of ghrelin (a hormone that stimulates hunger) go up. This can make you feel hungrier, and hence you overeat and automatically choose foods that give you an instant 'kick' (typically high-GI carbs and sugary foods). Insulin and cortisol levels increase, causing the body to store energy as fat and making you feel hungrier. Cortisol, often called the 'stress hormone', increases significantly with lack of sleep. Not only does this cause increased heart rate, blood pressure, blood glucose, muscle tension and slower digestion, it also triggers a need for serotonin, a chemical produced by your body that affects your mood and appetite. When you have higher levels of cortisol and your body needs serotonin, you tend to crave carbohydrates and fats, which psychologically make you feel happy and satisfied. You can see how sleep deprivation can have a truly negative impact on your weight.

One of the key factors that influences weight gain is the amount of carbohydrates we consume. While some people are able to eat carbohydrates at every meal without much effect on their weight, other people's bodies cannot tolerate them as much and their weight is much more easily and significantly affected.

In my clinic, one main focus is to control carbohydrate intake, particularly among diabetics. When my patients start on their maintenance plan, we initially introduce just a few carbohydrates, like oats for breakfast, and more freedom in the choice of vegetables by reintroducing starchier vegetables, such as beetroot, carrots and onions. I take a blood sample and check the patient's HbA1c levels to monitor them. We gradually introduce more and more carbohydrates, which could be a potato at dinner and some fruit for snacks, depending on their choices and requirements. If their bloods remain in the non-diabetic range, it means that the person is able to tolerate that level of carbohydrates and the diet plan can continue with them included. If there is any concern, we can reduce the carbohydrates again until we find a balance where both the weight and HbA1c remain stable.

Age also plays an important role in weight maintenance. If a person aged 50 is maintaining their weight with their current diet and lifestyle, the same diet and lifestyle may need to be reviewed in ten years' time in order to help them maintain their weight. As we age, our body composition changes and our level and intensity of activity generally reduces, so we do not require as many calories as we did when we were younger.

While I cannot give you an exact plan for your maintenance diet without first meeting you, here's an idea of what a three-day sample meal maintenance plan could look like.

## Maintenance sample meal plan

|  | Day 1 | Day 2 | Day 3 |
|---|---|---|---|
| **Breakfast** | Frittata Breakfast Cups (p. 113); coffee with milk | Tropical Breakfast Smoothie (p. 114) | Cloud Bread with Smoked Salmon and Avocado (p. 105), herbal tea |
| **Snack** | Finn Crisp Rolls with Cream Cheese (p. 125) | Mediterranean Dip with carrot and celery sticks (p. 213) | Aubergine Pizzas (p. 206) |
| **Lunch** | Buffalo Chicken Wrap Pizza (p. 131) | Green Lentil and Pomegranate Molasses Salad (p. 126) | Tomato and Bean Soup (p. 139) |
| **Snack** | Creamy Vegetable Soup (p. 138) | Celeriac and Cabbage Slaw (p. 146) on wholemeal crackers | Yuk Sung (p. 159) |
| **Dinner** | Moussaka (p. 181) | Vegetarian Lasagne (p. 190); rocket and cherry tomato salad | Cape Malay-style Fish Curry (p. 186), small glass of red wine |
| **Snack** | Creamy Cowberry and Quark Dessert (p. 223) | Small bag of popcorn | Chilled Chocolate and Avocado Mousse (p. 220) |

# THE RECIPES

# Introduction

In my opinion, no diet can be healthy without vegetables. As you'll see from my recipes, vegetables make up the bulk of what you eat during the diet. I believe that if this forms a new habit, you will not struggle to maintain your weight and you will manage to keep your diabetes away. Many people eat some vegetables at dinnertime, but you will need to have vegetables twice a day to reach the required amount of 700g–800g every day. Although it sounds like a lot, you can easily reach this total by having a good-sized bowl of homemade soup at lunchtime and a plate full of vegetables as a stir-fry, vegetable curry, vegetable bake, roasted vegetables, stuffed vegetables, vegetable slaw or a large salad at dinnertime – the possibilities are endless!

I love cooking, but don't always have time to cook from scratch. So, although fresh vegetables always taste best, if you are also struggling with time, you can choose pre-chopped, frozen or tinned vegetables. Food manufacturers have 'copped on' recently, with consumers becoming inter-ested in low-carbohydrate 'carbohydrate substitutes', such as courgetti (courgette made into spaghetti with a kitchen utensil called a spiralizer), cauliflower couscous or cauliflower rice (grated cauliflower, sometimes with seasonings). Both of these are widely available in most supermarkets, although they do taste much better when made from scratch!

Don't fall into the trap of thinking that sweet potatoes are better than ordinary white potatoes, or that 'gluten-free' products are automatically healthier or lower in carbohydrates – they might not be – so check the label or go online and look up the nutritional values. If you miss potatoes, try my Turnip Chips (see p. 202) or make mash with cauliflower.

Most of my recipes have been tried and tested in my clinics, and we have also included some new ideas, such as the Pilau Cauliflower Rice (see p. 201) and Cloud Bread (see p. 105).

When you are on Phase 1 or Phase 2, make sure you only choose recipes suitable for these phases as you are following a ketogenic diet. However, once you are doing Phase 3 or Maintenance, you can use any of the recipes and even expand on Phase 1 and Phase 2 by experimenting with different vegetables.

**Note: all the oven temperatures in my recipes are for a fan oven, so if you are using a conventional oven, increase the temperature by 20°C.**

Happy and healthy cooking!

## List 1 and 2 Vegetables
## for VLCKD – Phases 1 and 2

| List 1 – Choose More Often | List 2 – Choose Sparingly |
| --- | --- |
| Asparagus | Aubergine |
| Beansprouts | Brussels sprouts |
| Broccoli | Celeriac |
| Cabbage | French beans |
| Cauliflower | Leek |
| Celery | Red cabbage |
| Chicory | Red and yellow peppers |
| Chinese cabbage | Swiss chard |
| Courgette | Tomato |
| Cucumber | Turnip |
| Fennel | |
| Gherkins | |
| Green pepper | |
| Kale | |
| Lettuce (all types) | |
| Mushrooms (all types) | |
| Pak choi | |
| Radish | |
| Scallion | |
| Spinach | |
| Watercress | |
| Rocket | |

## Recommended Cheeses
## for Phases 2, 3 and Maintenance

Cheese can be used as an alternative source of protein from Phase 2 onwards, which means that you could have cheese instead of fish, meat, eggs or poultry. Unfortunately, if eaten frequently, weight loss can be hindered by the sugar in milk (typically higher in softer cheeses than harder cheeses) and by the fat content of cheese. Here is a list of the most commonly used cheeses and suggested portions.

| Cheese Variety | Portion for Phase 2, 3 or Maintenance Dinner | Portion for Phase 3 or Maintenance lunch |
|---|---|---|
| Red Cheddar | 40g | 20g |
| Reduced-fat red Cheddar | 60g | 30g |
| White Cheddar | 40g | 20g |
| Half-fat mozzarella | 100g | 50g |
| Full-fat mozzarella | 60g | 30g |
| Feta | 60g | 30g |
| Light feta | 100g | 50g |
| Edam | 50g | 25g |
| Brie | 50g | 25g |
| Camembert | 60g | 30g |
| Emmental | 50g | 25g |
| Parmesan | 40g | 25g |
| Roquefort | 50g | 30g |
| Goats' cheese | 50g | 25g |
| Gruyère | 40g | 20g |
| Mascarpone | 40g | 20g |
| Ricotta | 120g | 60g |
| Stilton | 100g | 50g |
| Full-fat cottage cheese | 180g | 90g |
| Light cottage cheese | 200g | 100g |

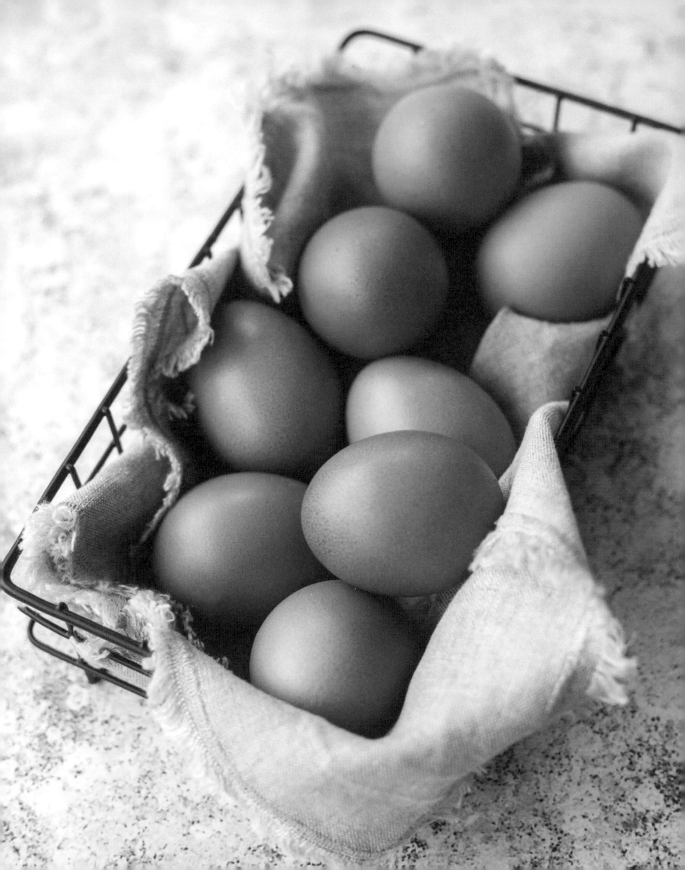

# BREAKFAST

# Eurodiet omelette

All of my patients know how passionate I am about vegetables, especially the greens. I strongly believe that if we all ate more of them, we would be in better health. Most of the people I meet in my clinics have vegetables typically just at dinnertime, and this is one of the first things they change when starting on the diet. Nothing stops you from having vegetables at breakfast – if asparagus isn't your favourite or you think it takes too long to cook it, try spinach instead. This recipe is suitable for breakfast, lunch or dinner.

— 2 Laktolight sachets
— 2 Eurodiet omelette sachets
— spray oil
— 8 baby asparagus spears
— mixed dried or fresh herbs and spices, such as chopped fresh chilli and parsley
— freshly ground black pepper

## HOW TO PREPARE

1 Fill the shaker with 200ml of water. Add the Laktolight sachets, close the lid and shake.
2 Empty the omelette sachets into the shaker. Close the lid and shake again, mixing well. Set aside.
3 Heat a grill pan. Coat it with spray oil and press the asparagus spears against it, cooking them gently and giving them some colour. Set aside, keeping them warm.
4 Heat a large non-stick pan over a low heat. Spray some oil on it, then pour in the omelette mixture, spreading it evenly, and sprinkle with your dried or fresh herbs and spices.
5 Once the omelette has set, carefully turn it over. Check to see that both sides are cooked. Add the asparagus over one half, then fold it over. Season with black pepper and serve warm.

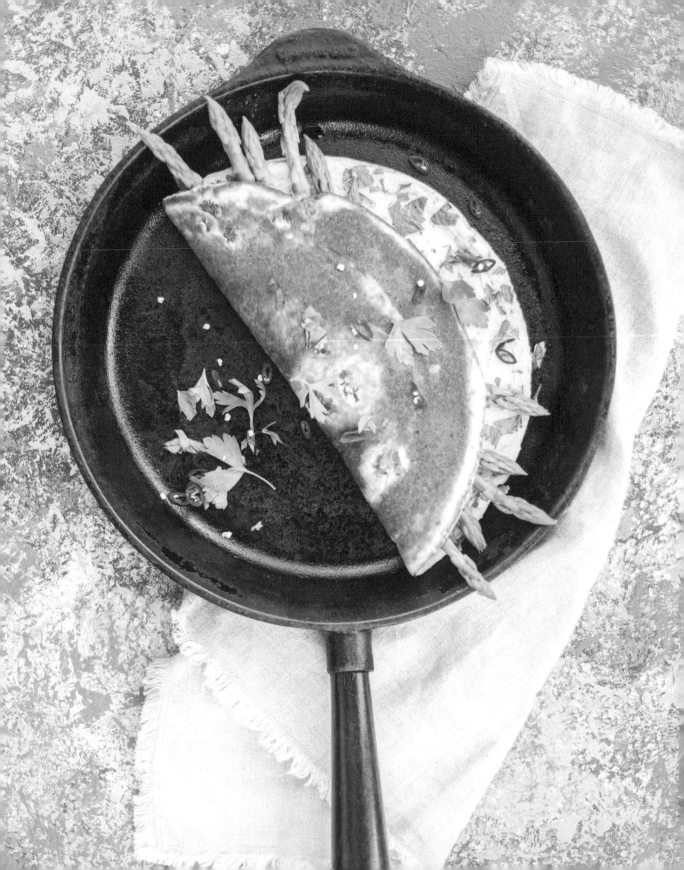

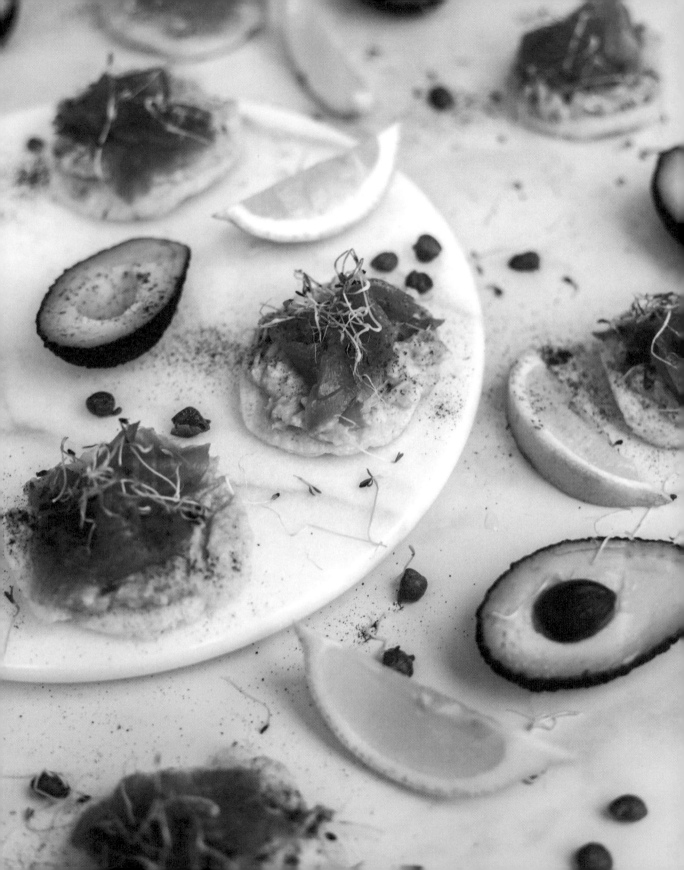

# Cloud bread with smoked salmon and avocado

MAINTENANCE | SERVES 4

Smoked salmon and avocado have become a big hit recently. They are both good for you in their own ways, but they are not low in calories. Most people have them with brown bread, which adds both carbohydrates and calories to the meal. These cloud 'breads' are a great substitute. Make them the night before and leave to cool overnight, uncovered. Serve on their own for breakfast, or with a bowl of soup or salad for lunch.

— spray oil
— 4 eggs
— 60g plain or seasoned light cream cheese
— ½ tsp cream of tartar
— pinch of freshly ground black pepper
— 1 large ripe avocado
— 120g smoked salmon
— 40g alfalfa
— capers (optional)
— squeeze of lemon juice, to serve

HOW TO PREPARE

1 Preheat the oven to 130°C.
2 Line a large baking tray with non-stick baking paper and spray it lightly with spray oil.
3 Separate the egg whites from the yolks. Place the egg whites in a large mixing bowl. Beat them with an electric hand whisk until they are white and foamy but not grainy. They should be stiff enough not to move if you tilt the bowl.
4 Place the cream cheese and egg yolks in another mixing bowl. Add the cream of tartar and whisk together until frothy.
5 Carefully fold the egg whites into the cream cheese mixture. Try to avoid the mixtures losing their frothiness.
6 Using a tablespoon, measure out 16 portions straight onto the prepared baking tray. Discard any runny mixture, as only the 'fluffy' mixture will work. Sprinkle with freshly ground black pepper.
7 Carefully place the tray into the oven. Bake for approximately 20 minutes, until the 'breads' start to get some colour. Remove from the oven and set aside to cool overnight.
8 When ready to serve, mash the avocado with a fork and spread it over the breads. Add some sliced smoked salmon and garnish with alfalfa and capers (if using). Squeeze over some lemon juice, if desired. Serve immediately, as the bread will become soggy and the avocado will start to turn brown.

# Eurodiet porridge with stewed rhubarb

PHASE 1 ONWARDS | SERVES 1

This porridge has some oat flakes in it, so the consistency is very similar to regular porridge cooked in milk. Most people find it sweet enough without toppings such as fruit and honey, but you can add stewed rhubarb for more bulk. The reason why this porridge works on the diet is that it has only one-third of the carbohydrates and four times more protein than a serving of regular porridge oats! As you only need a bowl, a spoon and boiled water, it's ideal for those mornings on the go or even when travelling.

Many people mistakenly think of rhubarb as a fruit, but it's actually a brilliant vegetable to use during the diet. Rhubarb is an ideal way to add more vegetable fibre to your breakfast and you can have the leftovers as a 'free' snack any time of the day, as this makes more than you'll need for one serving of porridge.

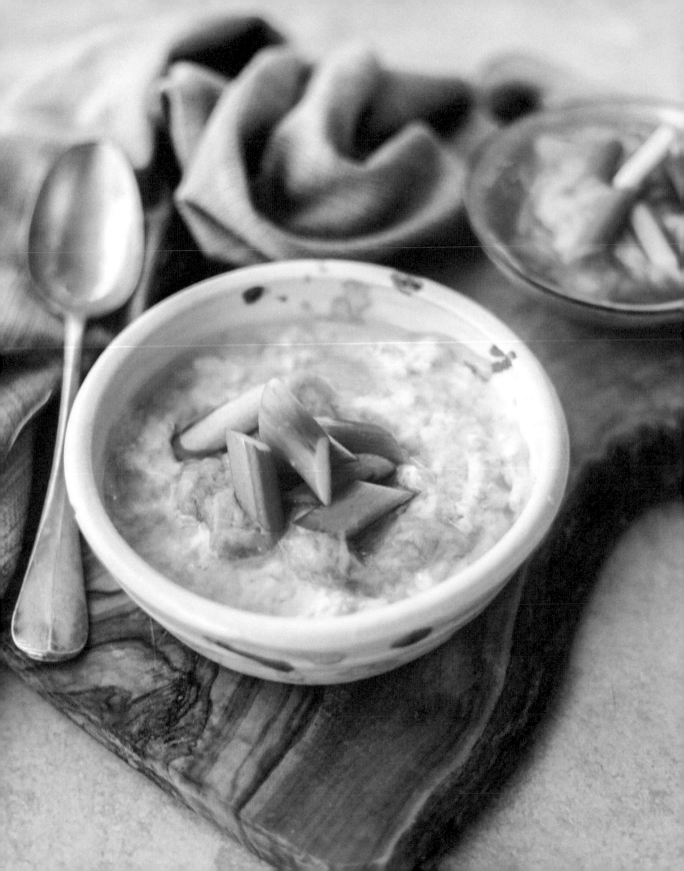

- 1 Eurodiet porridge sachet
- 1 Laktolight sachet

**FOR THE STEWED RHUBARB:**
- 1 bunch of rhubarb, chopped (usually about 5 stalks, size varying throughout season)
- xylitol, to taste
- pinch of ground cinnamon (optional)

## HOW TO PREPARE

1 Place the chopped rhubarb in a saucepan. Add just enough water to cover. Bring it to the boil, then reduce the heat and simmer for 5 minutes without a lid to allow the excess water to evaporate.

2 Remove from the heat and sweeten to taste with xylitol and a pinch of cinnamon (if using).

3 Empty the sachets of Eurodiet porridge and Laktolight into a cereal bowl. Mix well and gradually stir in 100ml of boiling water from the kettle.

4 Serve warm with some stewed rhubarb and/or a sprinkle of ground cinnamon.

# Eurodiet strawberry chia pudding

PHASE 1 ONWARDS | SERVES 1

HOW TO PREPARE

Chia seeds are a great source of good fibre and fats as well as some minerals, such as magnesium and calcium. These minerals are vital for healthy bones, and along with the good omega-3 fatty acids in the chia seeds, you will be getting a good start to your day. This pudding is a quick alternative to porridge, but rather than just having the smoothie, you get a more filling pudding out of it. Plus you can just grab the container and take it with you in the morning! It's also a great dessert.

— **2 tbsp whole chia seeds**
— **Eurodiet strawberry smoothie**

1 Prepare this breakfast the night before. Measure the chia seeds into a portable plastic container with a lid. Pour in the smoothie and stir well. Stir it once again before going to bed so that the seeds don't end up as one big clump, but rather start to form a gel-like mixture with the smoothie. Cover with a lid and leave in the fridge overnight.

# Eurodiet rice pudding

HOW TO PREPARE

This quick breakfast will keep you full for a long time. You can also have it as a protein source during Phase I after a dinner of vegetables, such as a stir-fry, as it contains the same amount of protein as five large eggs! The vanilla dessert has a lovely custard-like flavour, so many people find it very comforting. A similar dessert of rice and vanilla custard in the supermarket comes with approximately 25g of sugar, which is likely to turn into body fat although the product itself is labelled low-fat – a good example of why consumers need to be wary of misleading food labelling. This is also a great dessert after a dinner of vegetables.

— **1 Eurodiet konjac rice sachet**
— **1 Laktolight sachet**
— **1 Eurodiet vanilla dessert sachet**
— **pinch of ground cinnamon (optional)**
— **cinnamon stick, to decorate (optional)**

1 Empty the contents of the rice sachet into a colander and rinse well under cold running water. Set aside to drain.
2 Measure 100ml of water into your shaker. Add the Laktolight sachet, close the lid and shake well.
3 Add the vanilla dessert sachet and close the lid. Shake well again to combine.
4 Place the rice in a microwave-proof cereal bowl. Pour in the vanilla dessert mixture and mix well.
5 Microwave at 900W for 1 minute. Add ground cinnamon to taste and decorate with a cinnamon stick (if using).

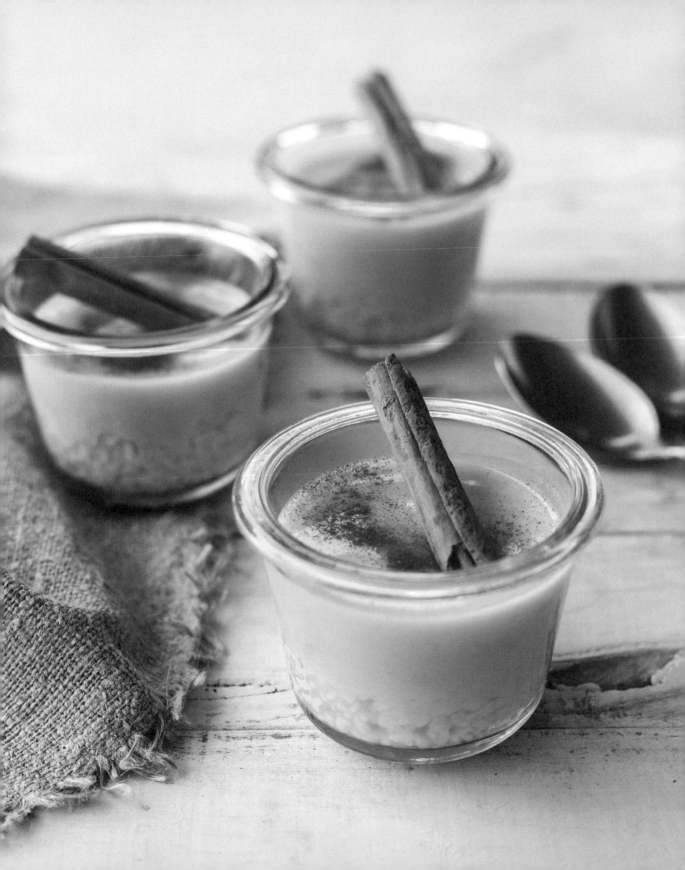

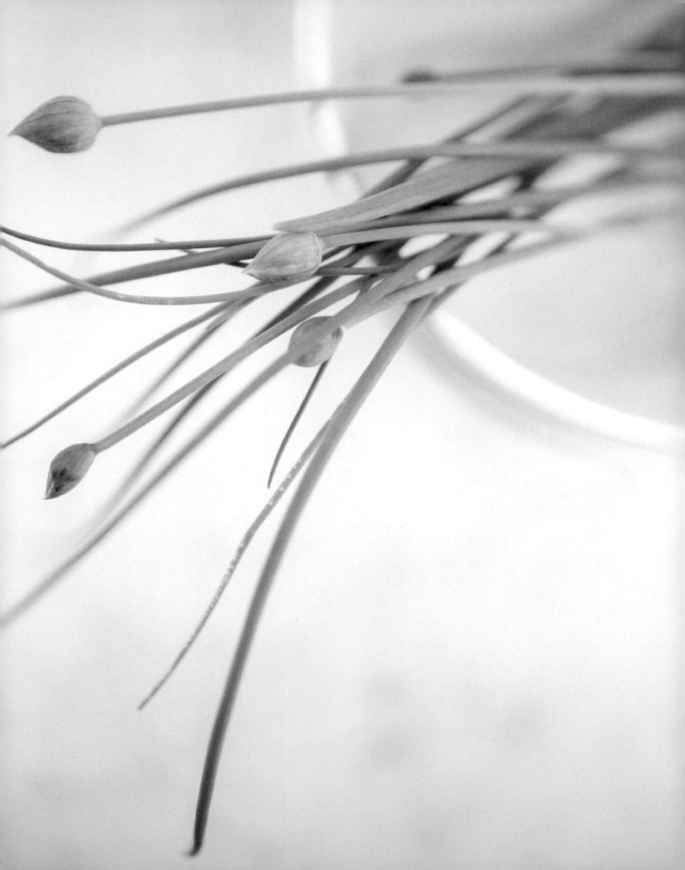

# Frittata breakfast cups

HOW TO PREPARE

Whisk these frittata cups up and have them cooking while grabbing your shower and getting ready. They taste just as nice when cold.

Eggs are an amazing source of nutrients. We now have a better understanding that the cholesterol that eggs contain not bad for you, but sadly the message has not spread. I still see people in my clinics who avoid eggs, while they are not concerned about having their toast with marmalade!

— **1 tsp butter**
— **3 slices of Black Forest ham, fat removed and cut into small pieces**
— **25g Salakis light sheep's milk cheese, crumbled**
— **5g fresh chives, finely chopped**
— **6 eggs**
— **freshly ground black pepper**

1  Preheat the oven to 160°C. Grease a 6-cup muffin tin with the butter.
2  Divide the ham pieces, cheese and chives between the muffin cups.
3  Crack the eggs into a mixing bowl with a spout, or use a jug. Whisk the eggs and black pepper together for 2–3 minutes.
4  Pour the whisked eggs evenly between the muffin cups. Cook in the oven for 12–15 minutes, until set. Serve warm or cold.

# Tropical breakfast smoothie

HOW TO PREPARE

Start your day right with this rejuvenating blend. Kefir contains beneficial yeast and bacteria, which have been studied for their numerous health benefits, from boosting your immunity to aiding digestion. Both mango and matcha green tea powder contain an incredible amount of antioxidants that help us battle the oxidative damage we are exposed to every single day. Aside from all these health benefits, it also tastes good!

— **100g frozen mango cubes or ½ medium fresh mango**
— **200ml kefir**
— **½ tsp matcha green tea powder**
— **a few drops of vanilla extract** (optional)

1  If using frozen mango, take the cubes out of the freezer 1–2 hours beforehand to defrost at room temperature or overnight in the fridge. If using fresh mango, just peel it and cut into cubes. Put into a NutriBullet blender.
2  Add the kefir, matcha powder and a few drops of vanilla extract (if using). Blend until smooth and serve chilled.

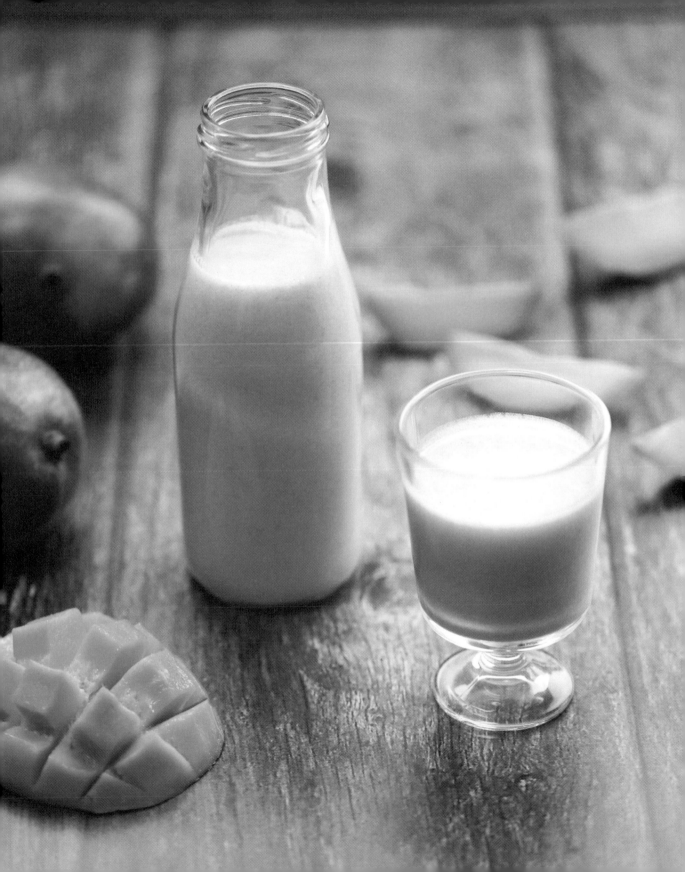

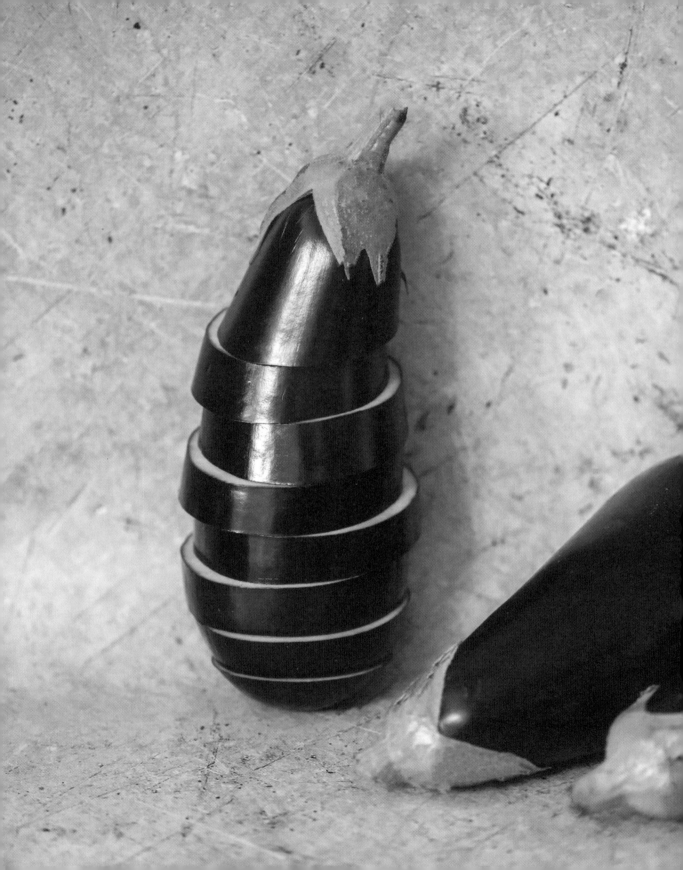

# LUNCH

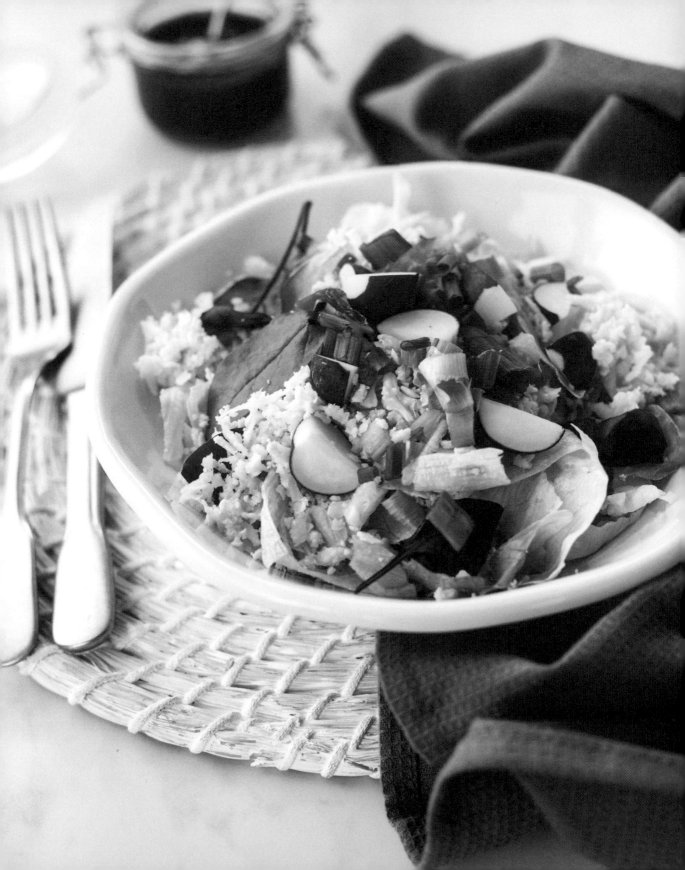

# Raw power salad with strawberry vinaigrette

PHASE 1 ONWARDS | SERVES 2–3

Raw foods have more nutrients than cooked foods, so they should be a staple part of our diet. Cooking destroys the vulnerable vitamin C that is abundant in fresh low-carbohydrate vegetables such as these radishes. Don't be afraid of trying the grated cauliflower, as it makes a great salad base. Serve this salad with a Eurodiet supplement in Phase 1, or with a portion of protein in Phase 2.

— 240g radishes, topped and tailed and cut into four wedges
— 1 medium-sized cauliflower, grated until the stem (discard the stem or use in soup)
— 1 small head of iceberg lettuce, chopped
— handful of mixed baby salad leaves
— 150ml good-quality apple cider vinegar
— 2 tbsp Eurodiet strawberry spread
— 1 tsp Herbamare salt
— freshly ground black pepper

## HOW TO PREPARE

1 Mix the radishes, grated cauliflower, iceberg lettuce and mixed leaves in a large salad bowl.
2 Mix the vinegar and Eurodiet strawberry spread in the shaker, then use this vinaigrette to dress the salad.
3 Season with Herbamare salt and freshly ground pepper and serve immediately.

# Eurodiet bread

This bread brings a lovely sense of normality to your diet. After all, isn't homemade brown bread and soup an all-time favourite lunch? Slice the loaf into 10 slices and freeze in groups of 2, as this bread does not keep well. Two slices of bread is a single portion.

— **spray oil, for greasing**
— **1 box of Eurodiet bread mix, containing 5 sachets of yeast and bread flour**
— **5 Laktolight sachets**
— **5 tsp psyllium husk (available in health food stores)**
— **1 tbsp milled flaxseeds**

## HOW TO PREPARE

1  Grease the inside of a 1lb bread loaf tin (20cm x 12cm) with spray oil.
2  Empty the contents of the bread mix, yeast and Laktolight sachets into a mixing bowl. Add the psyllium husk and mix well.
3  Put some cold water and boiled water into the shaker to make 250ml of very warm water. Add this to the dry ingredients and mix well with a spoon. Add the milled flaxseeds and knead the mixture for 3–4 minutes.
4  Tip the bread mix into the prepared loaf tin and even out the surface. This will make it easier for you to slice the bread into even slices once it is cooked.
5  Boil the kettle. Pour the boiled water in a medium-sized deep ovenproof dish and place the bread tin in the centre, taking care not to spill any water on the bread. This bain-marie helps the bread to rise. Cover with a clean towel and set aside for 1 hour.
6  Preheat the oven to 180°C.
7  Remove the loaf tin from the water and bake in the middle of the oven for 35 minutes. Allow to cool before slicing.

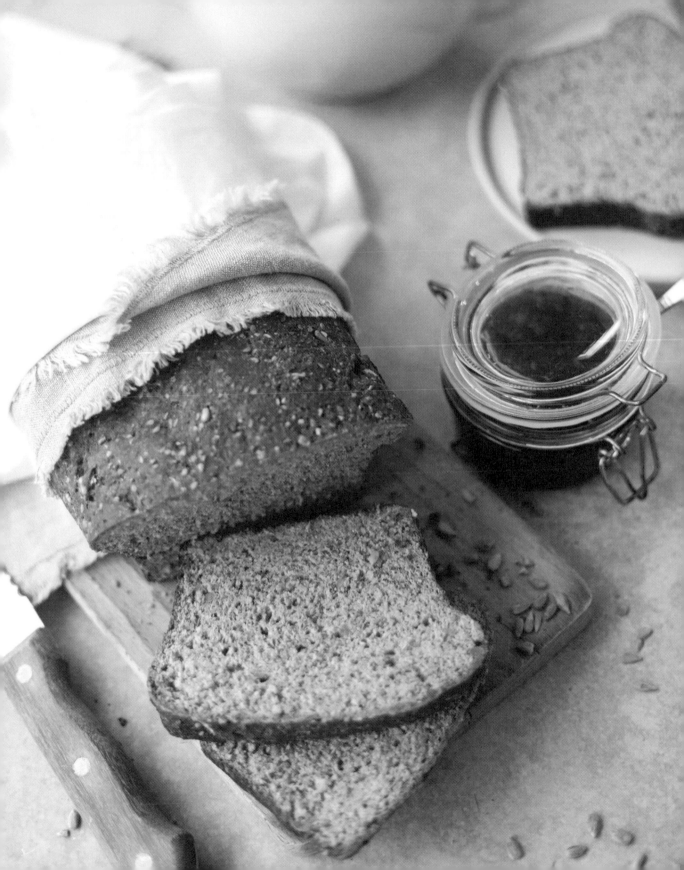

# Eurodiet pasta salad with pesto

PHASE 1 ONWARDS | SERVES 2

Fresh pesto makes this pasta dish come alive, and luckily most supermarkets now stock it. Fresh garlic is an excellent source of allicin, which has been getting a lot of good press for its health-enhancing properties.

— 2 servings of Eurodiet pasta
— 60g flavoured light soft cheese, such as Philadelphia Garlic and Herbs
— 2 tbsp fresh green pesto
— 1 courgette, spiralized or very thinly sliced
— 2 garlic cloves, crushed
— ½ tsp Herbamare salt
— 300g washed mixed leaves
— 10g pine nuts
— black and green fresh basil leaves, to garnish

## HOW TO PREPARE

1 Cook the pasta as instructed on the packet and drain well. Transfer to a large bowl and add the pesto and soft cheese. Fold in the courgette and garlic and season with the Herbamare salt. Serve warm over a bed of mixed leaves. Scatter over the pine nuts and garnish with the fresh basil leaves.

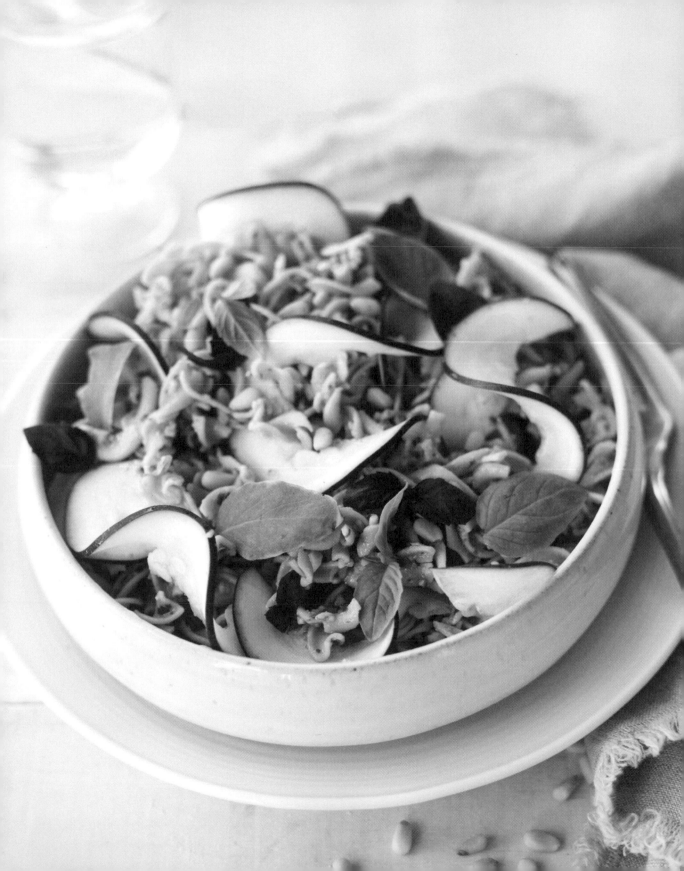

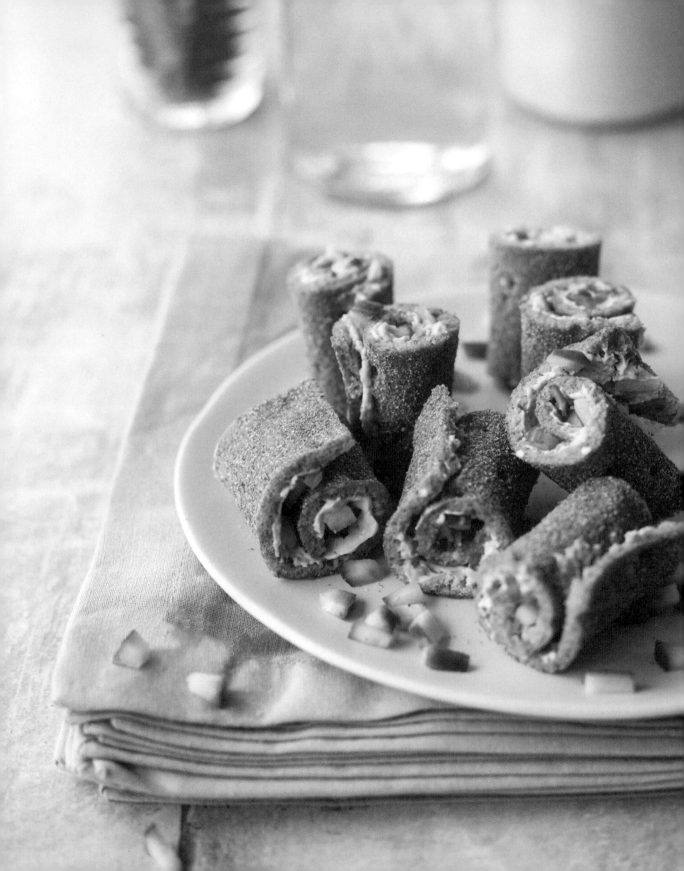

# Finn Crisp rolls with cream cheese

PHASE 3 ONWARDS | SERVES 2

HOW TO PREPARE

These rye crackers have an exceptional amount of fibre. They are a staple part of the Finnish diet, but you can get them in Ireland in some well-stocked health food shops and supermarkets. Add a luxurious feel to your everyday lunch by making these rolls or serve them for party guests. They get soggy rather fast after filling, so they are best served without delay.

— **8 Finn Crisp original sourdough rye thins**
— **80g light flavoured soft cheese, such as sweet chilli**
— **1 tbsp very finely chopped cucumber or very finely chopped fresh red chilli**

1 Pour some cold water into a deep dish. Dip each cracker in the water for a few seconds, until fully soaked.
2 Lay the soaked crackers side by side on a chopping board, leaving the rough side facing upwards. Cover with cling film and leave to stand for 12–15 minutes.
3 Meanwhile, cut a 5cm piece of cucumber. Cut it in half lengthways and remove the watery, seedy middle section. Cut the remaining cucumber into very small pieces. Alternatively, remove the seeds from a chilli and cut it into very small pieces.
4 Once the crackers are ready for rolling, start filling each one with cream cheese and the cucumber or chilli. Carefully roll each crispbread and seal the end by pressing gently with some more filling. Serve at lunchtime with a bowl of soup.

# Green lentil and pomegranate molasses salad

MAINTENANCE | SERVES 4–6

I got this recipe idea from a dear friend and colleague and it has never failed to satisfy me. Lentils and other legumes should become a staple in your maintenance diet as an alternative protein source, but they need to be omitted during the initial stages due to their carbohydrate content. They are rather flavourless on their own, so they can really benefit from all these herbs and spices. The real secret to this recipe is the right pomegranate molasses – look for the authentic one in shops that sell other typical Middle Eastern food.

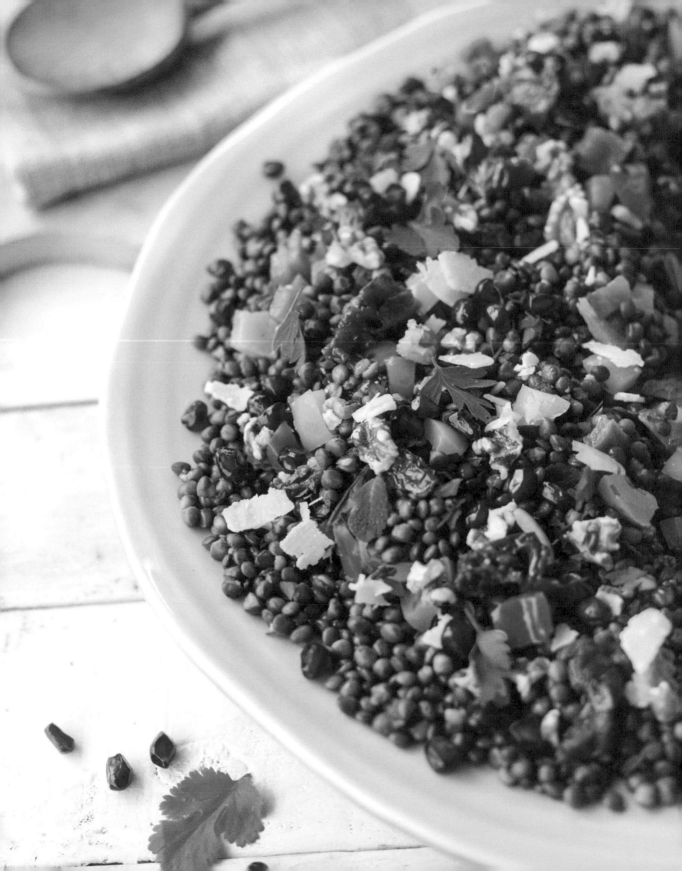

- 1.2kg/3 tins of green lentils (750g net weight)
- 2 tbsp olive oil
- 1 onion, finely chopped
- 2 garlic cloves, crushed
- 3 peppers, mixed colours, finely chopped
- 285g jar of sun-dried tomatoes in oil (net weight 140g), drained well on kitchen paper
- 35g fresh flat-leaf parsley leaves, roughly chopped
- 20g fresh mint, stems removed and leaves roughly chopped
- 30g walnuts, roughly chopped
- 80g pomegranate seeds
- 60g Parmesan cheese flakes

**FOR THE SALAD DRESSING:**
- 1 lemon, zest and juice
- 2 tbsp good-quality pomegranate molasses
- 1–2 tsp Maldon sea salt
- freshly ground pepper

## HOW TO PREPARE

1 Rinse the lentils in a colander under cold running water, taking care not to mush them. Set aside to drain well.

2 Heat the olive oil in large non-stick pan. Sauté the onion and garlic first for 3 minutes, then add the peppers. Cook for another 5 minutes, until softened but still crunchy. Remove the cooked vegetables from the pan and set aside to cool.

3 While the vegetables are cooking, cut the drained sun-dried tomatoes into small pieces using kitchen scissors. Place the drained lentils and sun-dried tomatoes in a large bowl. Add the herbs and walnuts and stir gently to combine.

4 Make the dressing by putting the lemon zest and juice into a bowl. Mix in with the pomegranate molasses, salt and pepper. Stir well and pour over the salad, gently tossing to combine.

5 To serve, sprinkle the salad with the pomegranate seeds and Parmesan cheese flakes.

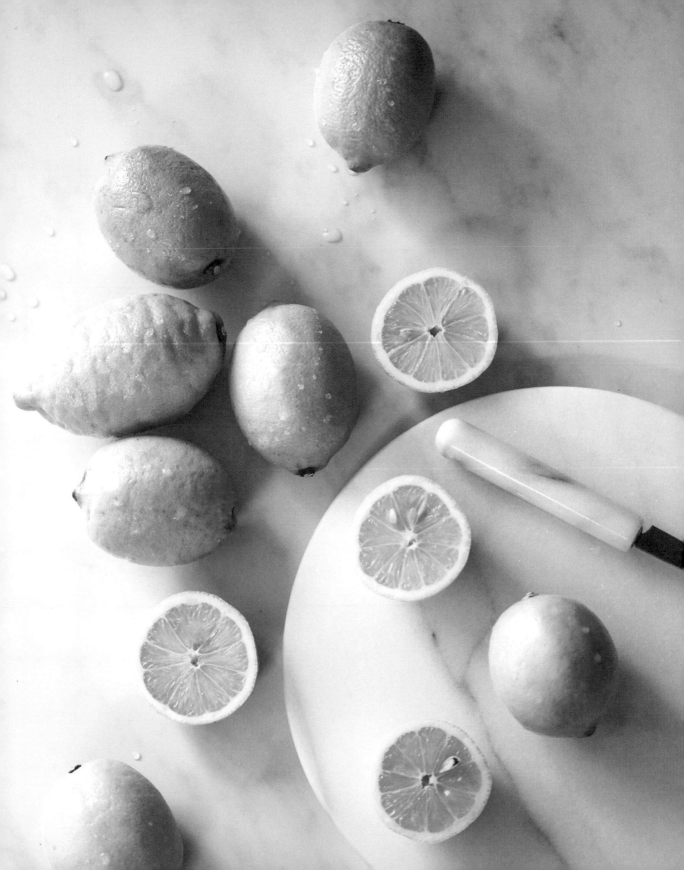

# Warm chicken and coconut salad

PHASE 3 ONWARDS | SERVES 4

This is a tasty salad that introduces fruit into the diet, so it's a great Phase 3 recipe. Fruit contains fructose, and although this is a 'natural' sugar, it still can affect your blood sugar readings, so you need to have it in moderation.

— **10 tbsp desiccated coconut, scattered on a large plate**
— **12 mini chicken fillets, white parts removed**
— **2 eggs, beaten**
— **Herbamare salt**
— **2 baby gem lettuces, shredded**
— **250g baby spinach**
— **1 red pepper, chopped**
— **1 orange pepper, chopped**
— **1 small fresh pineapple, peeled and cut into chunks**
— **60ml avocado oil**

## HOW TO PREPARE

1 Preheat the oven to 180°C. Cover a baking tray with foil.
2 Scatter the desiccated coconut on a large plate. Dip the chicken fillets in the beaten egg, then coat in the coconut.
3 Place the fillets on the prepared tray and season lightly with Herbamare salt. Bake in the oven for 15–20 minutes, until the chicken is cooked through and the coconut has started taking on some colour.
4 While the chicken is cooking, arrange the salad vegetables between four serving plates. Place the lettuce and spinach leaves at the bottom, then add the peppers and pineapple on top.
5 To serve, place 3 cooked chicken mini fillets on top of each salad and drizzle with the avocado oil.

# Buffalo chicken wrap pizza

Give yourself a break from soup at lunchtime and try this tasty wrap pizza instead. Have some vegetables at breakfast or snack on some crudités and Mediterranean vegetable dip (page 213) before your lunch to get your daily fibre. Look for wholemeal wraps with as little added starches as possible.

— 2 wholemeal wraps
— 2–3 tbsp Frank's RedHot Buffalo Wings Sauce
— 1 x 140g packet of cooked roast chicken breast, diced small or already torn
— 6 tbsp Mutti pizza sauce (available in tins in large supermarkets)
— 60g grated mozzarella and Cheddar cheese mixture
— 30g blue cheese, crumbled

## HOW TO PREPARE

1 Preheat the oven to 180°C.
2 Place the wraps on two separate pizza trays or one large baking tray.
3 In a small bowl, mix the buffalo wing sauce with the chicken pieces.
4 Spread the pizza sauce evenly over the two wraps. Scatter over the chicken pieces, then both cheeses.
5 Cook in the hot oven for approximately 8 minutes, until the cheese has melted and the chicken is hot.

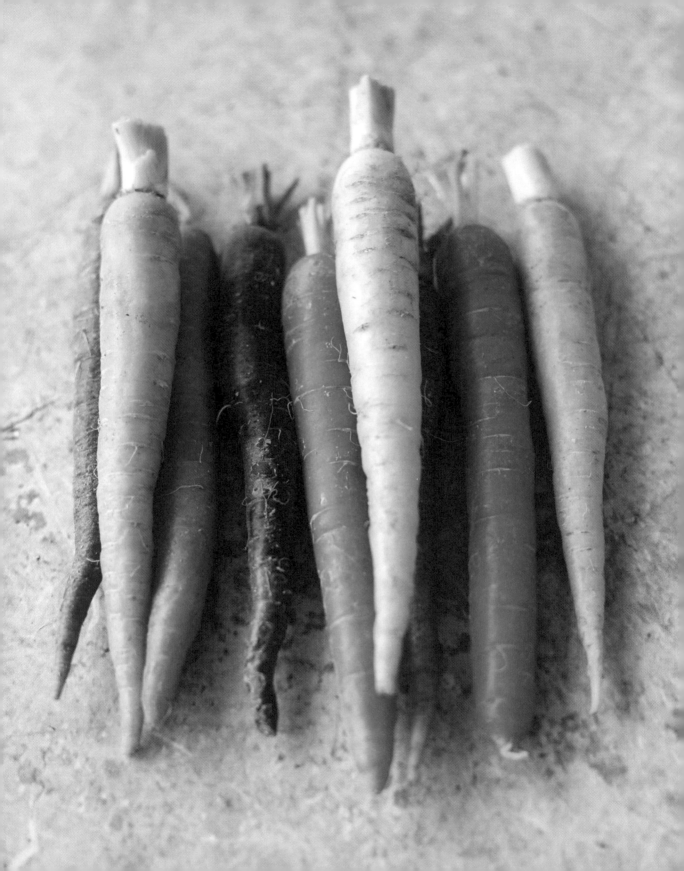

# SOUPS AND SALADS

# Asparagus and blue cheese soup

PHASE 1 ONWARDS | SERVES 3

Asparagus is beautiful and plentiful when it's in season. The Irish season starts in early May, when the delicate buds are at their very best. If you are looking for asparagus at a different time of the year, avoid getting 'woody' asparagus for this soup, as it will be very stringy and bitter.

— 1 chicken stock cube
— 1 tbsp olive oil
— 1 leek, white part only, washed and chopped
— 4 garlic cloves, crushed
— 25 medium-sized asparagus spears, chopped
  30g blue cheese

## HOW TO PREPARE

1 Dissolve the chicken stock cube in 850ml of boiling water.
2 Heat the oil in a saucepan. Add the leek and garlic and sauté until soft. Add the asparagus and pour in the stock. Bring to the boil, then reduce the heat and simmer for 30 minutes, until the asparagus is soft.
3 Add the blue cheese and blend for a smooth consistency.

# Cauliflower and celery soup with spices

PHASE 1 ONWARDS | SERVES 6–8

This Indian spiced soup is lovely and thick thanks to the cauliflower. Madras curry powder and the fresh chilli add a nice kick, but feel free to leave out the chilli and use a milder curry blend instead, such as korma. You should find both of these in the spice section of any large supermarket.

— 1 tbsp vegetable bouillon
— 1 tbsp coconut oil
— 4 garlic cloves, crushed
— 1–2cm piece of fresh red chilli, deseeded and finely chopped
— 1 small cauliflower, chopped
— 1 bunch of celery, chopped
— 2 tsp ground cumin
— 2 tsp ground coriander
— 2 tsp Madras curry powder
— 1 tsp allspice
— 80ml full-fat coconut milk
— 3 tbsp chopped fresh coriander

## HOW TO PREPARE

1 Dissolve the vegetable bouillon in 1 litre of boiling water.
2 Heat the oil in a large saucepan. Add the garlic and chilli and sauté for 5 minutes. Add the cauliflower, celery, all the spices and the stock. Bring to the boil, then reduce the heat and simmer for 20 minutes, until the cauliflower and celery are soft.
3 Remove from the heat, then stir through the coconut milk and chopped coriander. Blend for a smooth consistency.

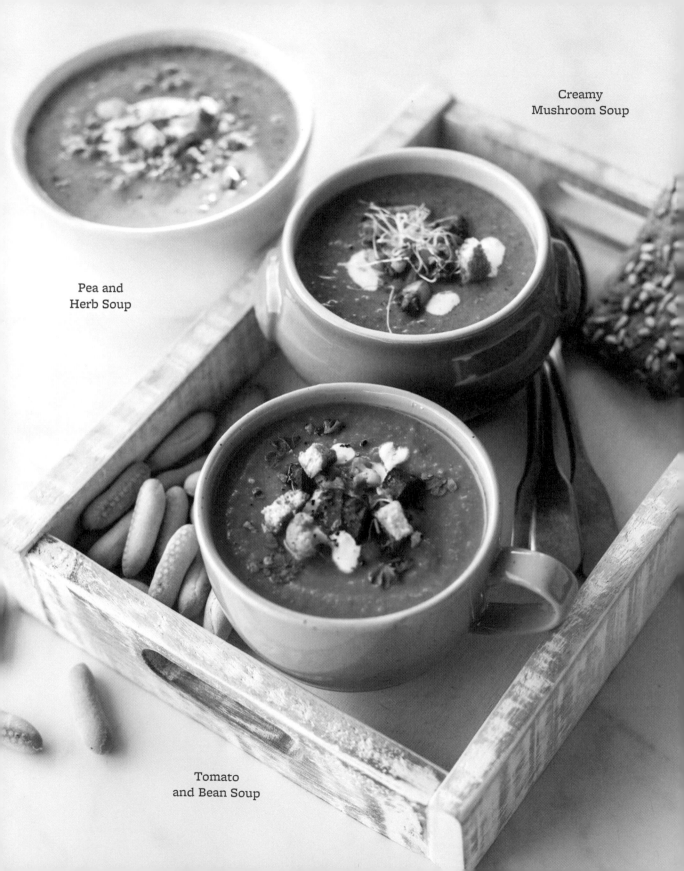

Creamy
Mushroom Soup

Pea and
Herb Soup

Tomato
and Bean Soup

# Chorizo and cauliflower soup

This soup will satisfy even the most fussy eaters, as chorizo adds that beautiful flavour. I find Cavabel cream cheese very flavoursome, even though it has more calories than other cream cheese brands – a little goes a long way. If you are using a different brand, make sure it's full-fat cream cheese. You can serve the soup with Eurodiet croutons in the initial phases and with some wholemeal bread once carbohydrates have been reintroduced.

— **2 Kallo tomato and herb stock cubes**
— **1 bunch of spring onions, finely chopped**
— **40g dry-cured chorizo, peeled if necessary and finely chopped**
— **900g caulilflower, chopped (approximately 2 small cauliflowers)**
— **400g tin of chopped tomatoes**
— **1 sprig of fresh rosemary**
— **50g Cavabel red pepper cream cheese (available in Lidl)**
— **chopped fresh flat-leaf parsley, to garnish**

## HOW TO PREPARE

1 Dissolve the stock cubes in 1 litre of boiling water.
2 Sauté the spring onions and chorizo together in large pan on a low heat for 5 minutes. Add the cauliflower, tinned tomatoes, rosemary sprig and stock. Bring to the boil, then reduce the heat and simmer for 25 minutes, until the cauliflower is soft.
3 Remove from the heat and discard the rosemary sprig and any large needles that have fallen off it. Add the cream cheese and blend with a hand-held blender until smooth. Ladle into bowls and garnish with chopped fresh parsley.

# Creamy vegetable soup

PHASE 1 ONWARDS | SERVES 3

This soup has become a staple for many of my patients. Even children find it pleasant, which is a huge benefit considering how some of my younger patients don't eat any vegetables before they start their journey with us. Soup keeps you fuller for longer than salads or vegetables alone. I recommend that people keep making soup during the maintenance phase. It's a great filler to have even just before going out for that well-deserved meal!

— **2 tsp vegetable bouillon**
— **1 tbsp olive oil**
— **1 leek, white part only washed and chopped**
— **4 garlic cloves, crushed**
— **1 orange pepper, chopped**
— **1 courgette, chopped**
— **60g ricotta cheese**
— **20 fresh basil leaves**

## HOW TO PREPARE

1. Dissolve the vegetable bouillon in 750ml of boiling water.
2. Heat the oil in a saucepan. Add the leek and garlic and sauté for 3 minutes. Add the pepper and courgette and cook for 5 minutes more. Pour in the stock and bring to the boil, then reduce the heat and simmer for 20 minutes.
3. Remove from the heat, then add the ricotta and basil. Blend until smooth and creamy.

# Tomato and bean soup

A simple, no-nonsense soup for those days when you want to make something quick and tasty. It works well as a base for those of you who like adding some extras. Rosemary and garlic are ideal, and you can choose just one variety of the tinned legumes if you prefer. Rinsing the tinned legumes is a must, as the brine contains a lot of sodium and thorough rinsing removes most of it.

— **2 vegetable stock cubes**

— **1 tbsp olive oil**

— **1 onion, diced**

— **4 celery sticks, chopped**

— **3 carrots, peeled and diced**

— **2 parsnips, peeled and diced**

— **2 x 400g tins of chopped tomatoes**

— **400g tin of chickpeas, drained and rinsed**

— **400g tin of butter beans, drained and rinsed**

### HOW TO PREPARE

1 Dissolve the stock cubes in 1 litre of boiling water.
2 Heat the oil in a large saucepan. Add the onion and cook for 3–5 minutes, until softened. Add the vegetables, tinned tomatoes, chickpeas, butter beans and stock and bring to the boil, then reduce the heat and simmer for 40 minutes. Blend if you prefer a smooth consistency.

# Pea and herb soup

Peas are too high in carbohydrates to use in bulk during the initial phases, but the small portion in this soup is fine. This soup tastes just as good with either basil or mint, and feel free to reduce the number of courgettes and add more peas once you are in the maintenance phase. You can even make a meal out of it by adding some leftover cooked ham if you have it.

You can serve the soup with Eurodiet croutons in the initial phases and with some wholemeal bread once carbohydrates have been reintroduced. You can also drizzle your serving with some fresh cream once you are in the maintenance phase.

— 1 tbsp vegetable bouillon

— 2 tbsp olive oil

— ½ large leek, washed and chopped finely

— 4 large courgettes, chopped

— 200g frozen peas

— 3-4 tbsp chopped fresh mint or basil, plus extra to garnish

— Eurodiet croutons, to garnish

— Herbamare salt and freshly ground black pepper

## HOW TO PREPARE

1. Dissolve the vegetable bouillon in 1 litre of boiling water.
2. Heat the oil in a large saucepan. Add the leek and sauté for a few minutes, then add the courgettes and frozen peas. Pour in the stock and bring to the boil, then reduce the heat and simmer for 15 minutes.
3. Remove from the heat and add the mint or basil. Blend for a smooth consistency. Add Herbamare salt and freshly ground black pepper to taste. Garnish with some extra chopped fresh mint or basil and add a few Eurodiet croutons if desired.

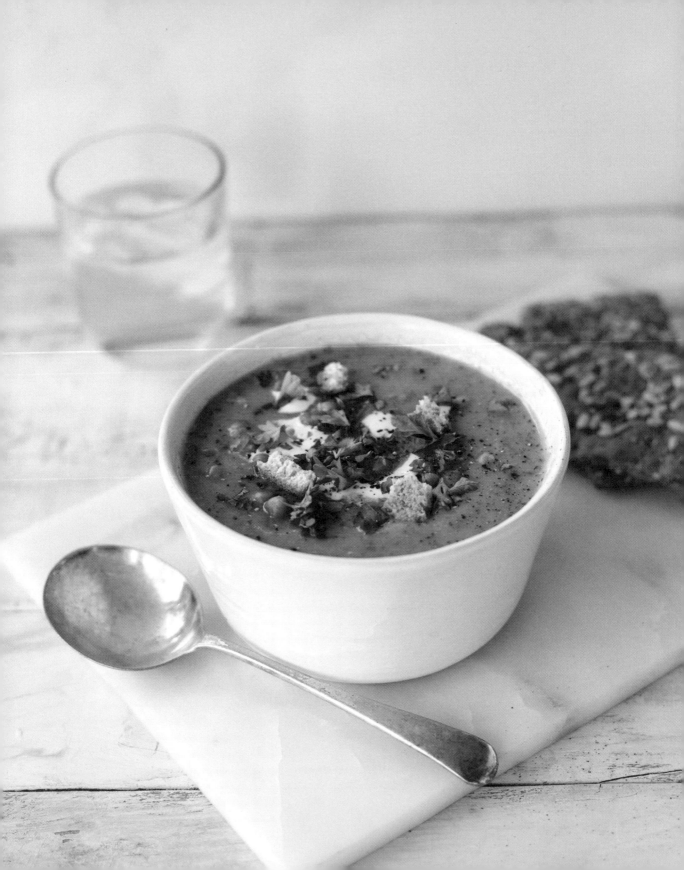

# Creamy mushroom soup

PHASE 1 ONWARDS | SERVES 3–4

Many of my patients love this mushroom soup. It's so easy to make that when you've made it once, you will remember the recipe the next time.

You can serve the soup with Eurodiet croutons in the initial phases and with some wholemeal bread once carbohydrates have been reintroduced. You can also drizzle your serving with some fresh cream once you are in the maintenance phase.

— 1½ mushroom stock cubes
— 600g mushrooms, washed and sliced
— 100g ricotta cheese
— 1 tbsp Dijon mustard
— alfalfa, to garnish

## HOW TO PREPARE

1 Dissolve the stock cubes in 700ml of boiling water.
2 Place the mushrooms and stock in a large saucepan. Bring to the boil, then reduce the heat and simmer for 20 minutes.
3 Remove from the heat and blend until smooth, then add the ricotta and mustard and blend well again. Garnish with a pinch of alfalfa.

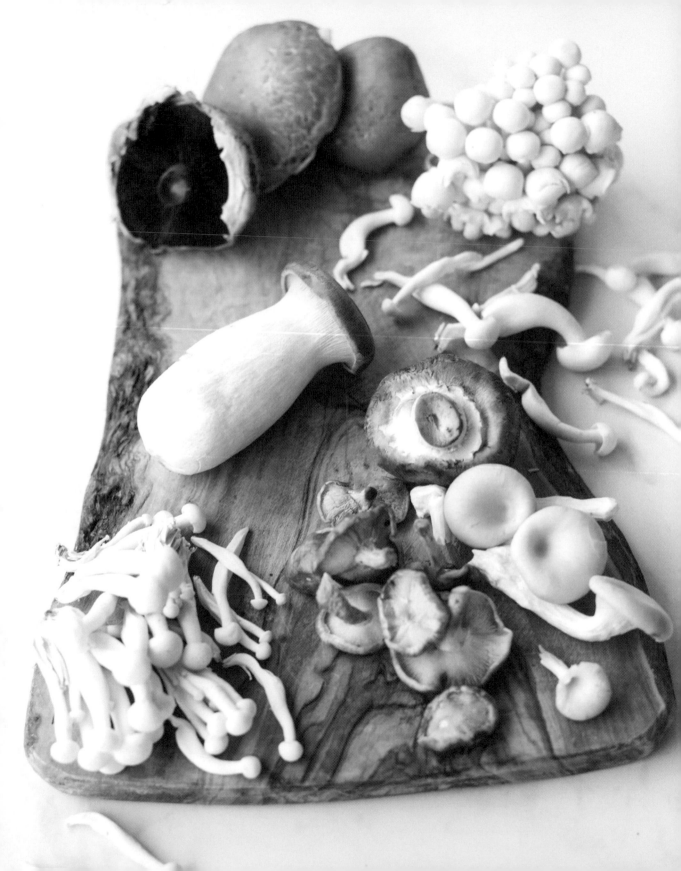

# Sweet potato and celeriac soup

MAINTENANCE | SERVES 8

HOW TO PREPARE

Sweet potato is exactly what the name implies: sweet. It contains more sugars than its humble rival, the regular potato. However, it gives this soup a satisfying sweetness, and when coupled with the lower-carbohydrate celeriac, it works very well. Celeriac is a vegetable that many people have never used. It has a rather unusual appearance, but it works well in many dishes. You can also try making chips out of it – just follow the recipe for Turnip Chips on p. 202, but instead of the Cajun seasoning, try Herbamare salt and some ground turmeric.

— 1 vegetable stock cube

— 1 tbsp olive oil

— 200g onions, chopped

— 2 tbsp peeled and grated fresh ginger

— 1 tbsp yellow curry paste

— 1kg sweet potatoes, peeled and cut into chunks

— 1kg celeriac, peeled and cut into chunks

— 1 lemongrass stalk, sliced into four lengthwise

1  Dissolve the stock cube in 1.5 litres of boiling water.
2  Heat the oil in a large pot. And the onions, ginger and yellow curry paste and sauté for 5 minutes on a low heat.
3  Add the sweet potatoes, celeriac and lemongrass, then pour in the stock. Bring the soup to the boil, then reduce the heat and simmer for 15 minutes, until the vegetables are soft.
4  Remove the lemongrass, then blend for a smooth consistency.

# Beetroot salad

Beetroots contain sugar, so you need to hold back from eating them during Phase 1 and Phase 2. You will surely appreciate it once you are able to reintroduce it from Phase 3 onwards. I love beetroot and it was a staple in my mother's kitchen so I use it a lot.

— **600g raw beetroot, peeled**
— **4 large green apples, peeled**
— **4 celery sticks, chopped**
— **4 tbsp orange juice**
— **2 tbsp olive oil**
— **2 tbsp balsamic vinegar**

HOW TO PREPARE

1 Grate the beetroot and apples into a large bowl. Add the celery and drizzle with the orange juice, oil and vinegar. Serve as part of a large green salad or as a side to a main course.

# Celeriac and cabbage slaw

PHASE 1 ONWARDS | SERVES 4

This salad was originally made years ago for a summertime recipe photo shoot in my house, but it has since remained one of the most popular salads in my clinics. You can serve it as a side to your main course, on its own or as part of a salad. Did you know that raw white cabbage has the same amount of vitamin C as grapefruit? Choose cabbages and celeriac that are approximately the same size, as this will make the consistency and flavour good.

— ½ white cabbage
— ½ red cabbage
— ½ celeriac, peeled

**FOR THE SALAD DRESSING:**
— 200g Hellmann's Lighter than Light mayonnaise
— 3 garlic cloves, crushed
— 1 large fresh red chilli, deseeded and very finely chopped
— juice of 1 lime
— zest of ½ lemon
— 10 fresh mint leaves, chopped
— 1 tsp Herbamare salt
— 1 tsp xylitol

## HOW TO PREPARE

1 Chop the cabbages and celeriac into pieces small enough to fit into the feed tube of your food processor. Use the food processor's grating blade to grate them. Empty the grated vegetables into a large container. Go through the vegetables to remove any large pieces that didn't grate well.
2 Mix all the salad dressing ingredients together in a large bowl, then mix in the grated vegetables.
3 Serve as part of a salad with green leaves or as a salad on its own.

# Chicken Caesar lettuce wrap

Many calorie-conscious people mistakenly order a chicken Caesar salad in restaurants. There are far more calories in a typical serving of this famous dish than there would be in something else that seems high-calorie, such as a steak and vegetables. But if you're a fan of the amazing flavour of the dressing, try this lower-calorie alternative way to enjoy the salad as a wrap instead. Don't bother with the reduced-calorie versions of the dressing – enjoy the real deal, but sparingly!

— 70g cooked chicken, diced small
— ½ bag Eurodiet Italian cheese and herb croutons, crumbled up
— 1 tbsp Caesar salad dressing (fresh varieties taste better!)
— 4 large leaves of cos lettuce
— 1 large plum tomato, cut into wedges and seeds removed

## HOW TO PREPARE

1 In a bowl, mix the chicken, croutons and salad dressing together in a bowl.
2 Cut out a square piece of greaseproof paper. Place two lettuce leaves on the paper and add the chicken and tomato. Place the other two leaves on top. Using the paper to help you, roll up the lettuce leaves into a wrap.

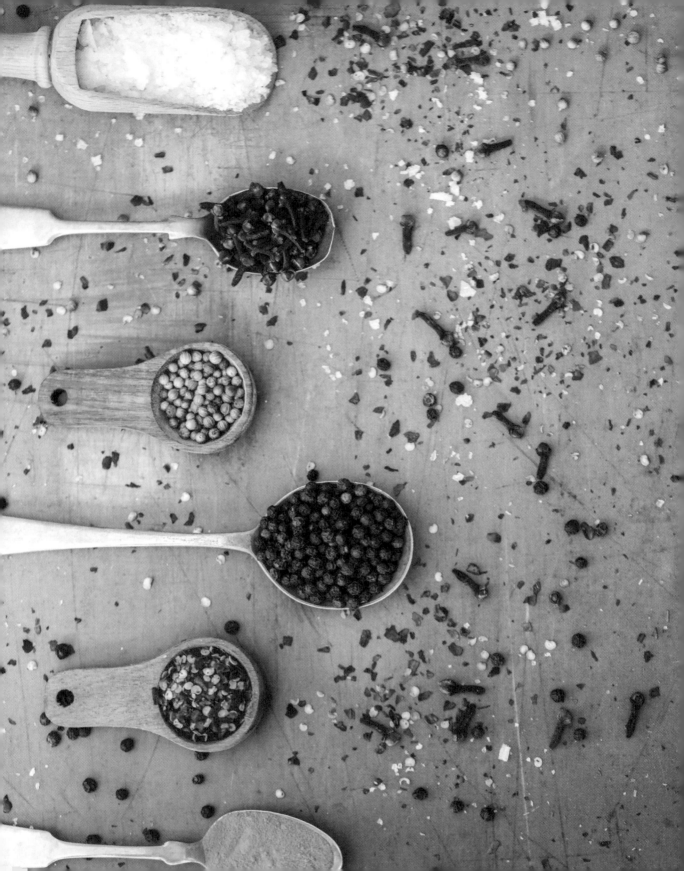

# DINNER

# Eurodiet egg fried rice

Don't be put off by the long list of ingredients! This dish is very fast to prepare, and once you have the right flavourings, it will taste great. Many soy sauces are a hidden source of sugar, so check the ingredients before buying.

— 1 Laktolight sachet
— 1 Eurodiet omelette sachet
— ½ tsp coconut oil
— 3 spring onions, chopped
— ½ tsp freshly grated ginger
— ½ tsp red curry paste
— 1 pak choi, finely chopped
— ½ orange pepper, thinly sliced
— 1 bag of Eurodiet konjac rice, rinsed well
— a few drops of brown rice vinegar
— a few drops of sugar-free soy sauce

## HOW TO PREPARE

1 Prepare the Eurodiet omelette mixture by measuring 100ml of cold water into the shaker and adding the Laktolight sachet. Shake this well, then add the omelette sachet, shake again and set aside.

2 Melt the oil in a non-stick pan. Add the spring onions, ginger and curry paste and sauté for 2 minutes. Add the pak choi and pepper and cook for an additional 2 minutes, then add the rice. Stir well and remove to a plate. Cover to keep warm.

3 Pour the omelette mixture into the same hot pan and immediately stir it around, making it the consistency of scrambled egg. Once cooked, add the rice and vegetable mixture back to the pan and quickly heat through. Season with the vinegar and soy sauce.

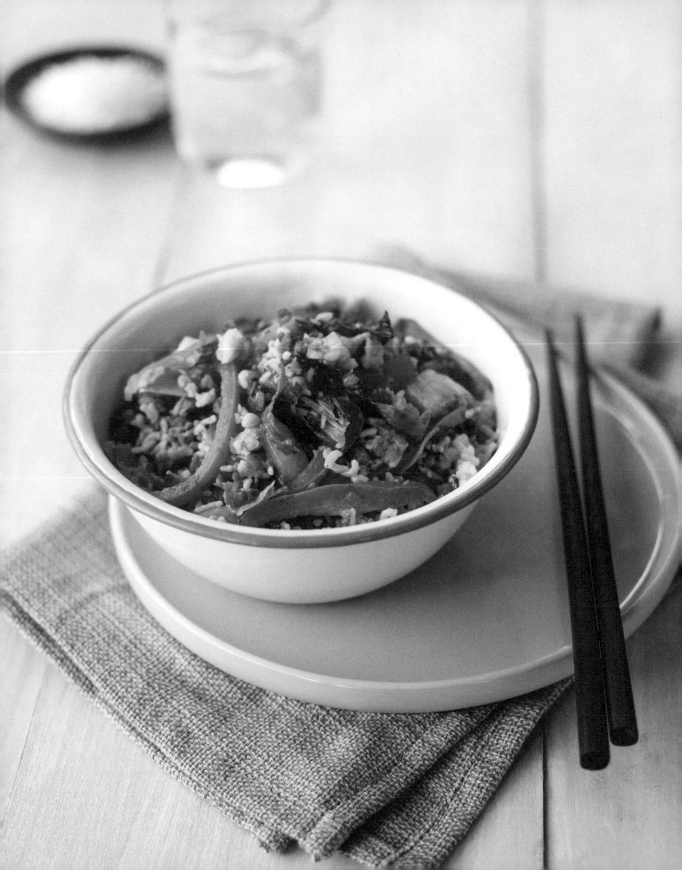

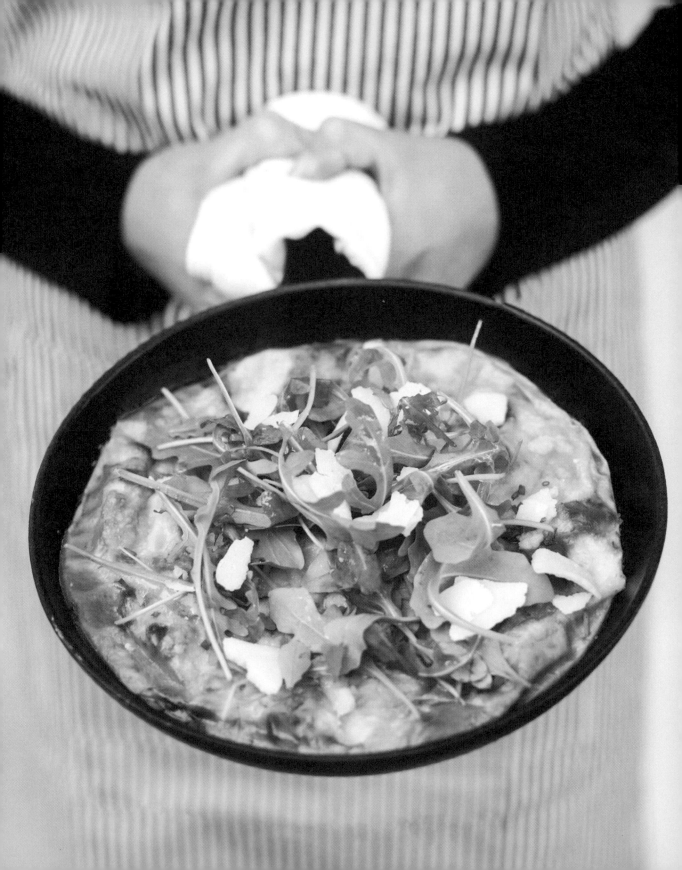

# Eurodiet frittata

PHASE 1 ONWARDS | SERVES 1

This is a quick weekday dinner that rises beautifully in the oven. I always aim to have 400g (almost 1lb) of vegetables at dinnertime, and this dinner is no exception. It would work just as well with many other vegetables, such as mushrooms and peppers, and with different salads on the side. You can also have it as your breakfast or lunch.

— 1 Laktolight sachet

— 1 Eurodiet omelette sachet

— 1 courgette, grated

— 1 small leek, washed and chopped

— spray oil

— chopped fresh herbs, such as chives and flat-leaf parsley (optional)

— handful of washed rocket

— 5g Parmesan cheese flakes

## HOW TO PREPARE

1 Preheat the oven to 180°C.

2 Prepare the Eurodiet omelette mixture by measuring 100ml of cold water into the shaker and adding the Laktolight sachet. Shake this well, then add the omelette sachet, shake again and set aside.

3 Sauté the courgette and leek with a few spritzes of spray oil in an ovenproof non-stick pan, allowing the excess water released from the vegetables to evaporate.

4 Pour the omelette mixture over the cooked vegetables and add the fresh herbs (if using). Place the pan in the oven and cook for 15 minutes.

5 Serve hot with the rocket on top and the Parmesan flakes scattered over.

# Eurodiet pizza

PHASE 1 ONWARDS | SERVES 2

Eurodiet flour contains 19g of protein per serving with only 3g carbohydrates! Although I've used only green peppers, you can have any of the suitable vegetables on this pizza – try asparagus, broccoli, mushrooms or fresh tomatoes. Try adding some Biona hot pepper sauce or Tabasco sauce to the pizza sauce and use jalapeño peppers and fresh chilli to get that fiery kick. During the maintenance phase you can be more liberal with your toppings and choose high-calorie extras such as blue cheese, olives or sun-dried tomatoes.

— **2 Laktolight sachets**
— **2 Eurodiet organic bread flour sachets**
— **2 Eurodiet yeast sachets**
— **2 tsp olive oil**
— **spray oil**
— **5 tbsp Mutti pizza sauce (or passata with some dried oregano added to it)**
— **1 green pepper, finely chopped**
— **60g Cheddar cheese, grated**
— **handful of rocket leaves**
— **mixed leaves, to serve as a side salad**

HOW TO PREPARE

1 Place the contents of the Laktolight and the Eurodiet bread flour and yeast sachets in a small heatproof bowl or a lunch box with a lid. Add the oil and mix well. Boil the kettle.

2 Using your shaker or a measuring jug, combine cold tap water with the boiled water to make 80ml of warm water. Add the warm water to the dry ingredients and knead the mixture for an even consistency. Make a dough ball using your hands and place in the centre of your heatproof bowl or lunch box.

3 Place a lid on the bowl or wrap your lunch box with foil. Place it in a large heatproof dish and add some weight over it (such as any heavier dish). Pour boiled water from the kettle into the large dish until it comes halfway up the sides of the smaller dish. Leave to rise for 1 hour.

4 Preheat the oven to 180°C.

5 Once the dough is ready, roll the dough into a circle on a piece of non-stick baking paper sprayed with spray oil. Spread the pizza sauce over the top, then add the pepper (or your vegetable of choice) and sprinkle with the cheese.

6 Place in the centre of the oven and bake for 25 minutes. Top with rocket leaves and serve with a side salad.

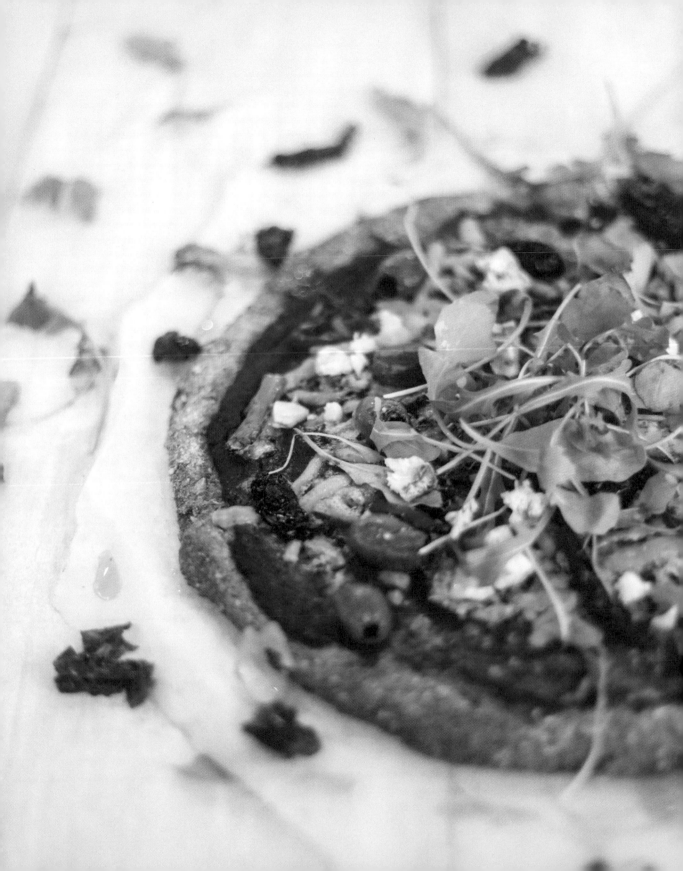

# Stuffed tomatoes

If you like to eat a lot of food and little calories, this is the recipe for you! These beautiful tomatoes will make everyone else jealous of your meal. The best thing is that they taste lovely and take minimal preparation time. You can even cook something else while they are in the oven.

— 4-6 large ripe tomatoes
— 1 Eurodiet vegetarian spicy spaghetti Bolognese packet
— ½ bag of Eurodiet konjac rice, rinsed well
— 1 tbsp Worcester sauce
— 1 tsp Biona hot pepper sauce or Tabasco
— handful of rocket leaves

## HOW TO PREPARE

1 Preheat the oven to 180°C.
2 Carefully remove the tops of the tomatoes using a small sharp knife. Set the tops aside. Using a spoon, scoop out the inside of each tomatoes, taking care not to break the skin. Place the tomatoes upright in an ovenproof dish, ready to be filled. Discard the insides of the tomatoes, or save for a soup.
3 Empty the contents of the vegetarian spicy spaghetti Bolognese packet and the rinsed konjac rice into a non-stick saucepan. Add 150ml of water, the Worcester sauce and hot pepper sauce and bring to the boil, then reduce the heat and simmer for 3–4 minutes, stirring occasionally.
4 Using a spoon, stuff the tomatoes with the Bolognese and rice mixture, then put the top of each tomato back on. Place in the centre of the oven and cook for 15 minutes, until the skin of the tomatoes is cooked. Serve with a handful of rocket leaves on the side.

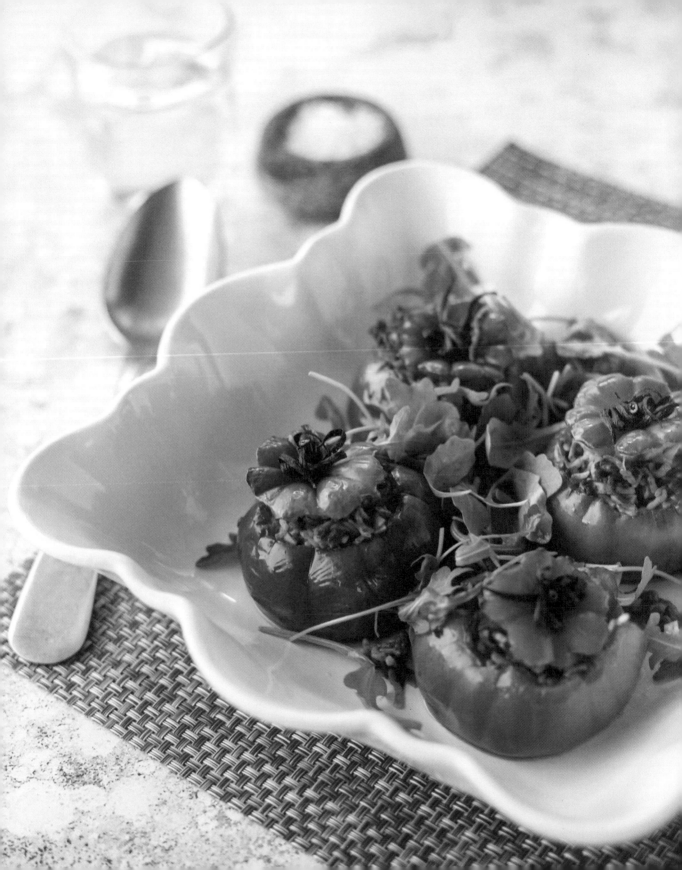

# Spicy chicken and vegetable casserole

Dieting doesn't seem like such an issue when you are able to have satisfying meals, such as this casserole. You're more likely to succeed when you get pleasure out of your food. People who develop better cooking skills during their journey are also more likely to do well during the maintenance phase.

— 20g butter
— 300g mini chicken fillets, cut into four pieces
— 80g leek, washed and chopped
— 3 celery stalks, chopped
— 1 large courgette, chopped
— 1 green pepper, chopped
— 230ml tomato passata
— 2 tsp Biona hot pepper sauce
— 2 tsp Worcester sauce
— ½ tsp Herbamare spicy salt
— 20g Cavabel red pepper cream cheese (available in Lidl)

## HOW TO PREPAPRE

1  Melt the butter in large, deep non-stick pan. Add the chicken pieces and cook until gently browned. Add all the chopped vegetables and cook over a low heat for 10 minutes, stirring occasionally. Add the passata, hot pepper sauce, Worcester sauce and Herbamare salt, then cover with a lid. Leave to simmer on a medium heat for 10 minutes, stirring occasionally.

2  Remove from the heat and add the cream cheese. Stir through to heat it. Serve hot with mashed cauliflower or a side of your choice.

# Yuk sung with spicy cabbage

This take on the classic yuk sung is a fantastic way to enjoy a restaurant-style meal with a fraction of the carbohydrates. It's also a nice meal to have with friends or at home with family on a Saturday night. Pork mince has a fabulous flavour in itself. You can substitute it with minced turkey or chicken, but it will most likely need more seasonings.

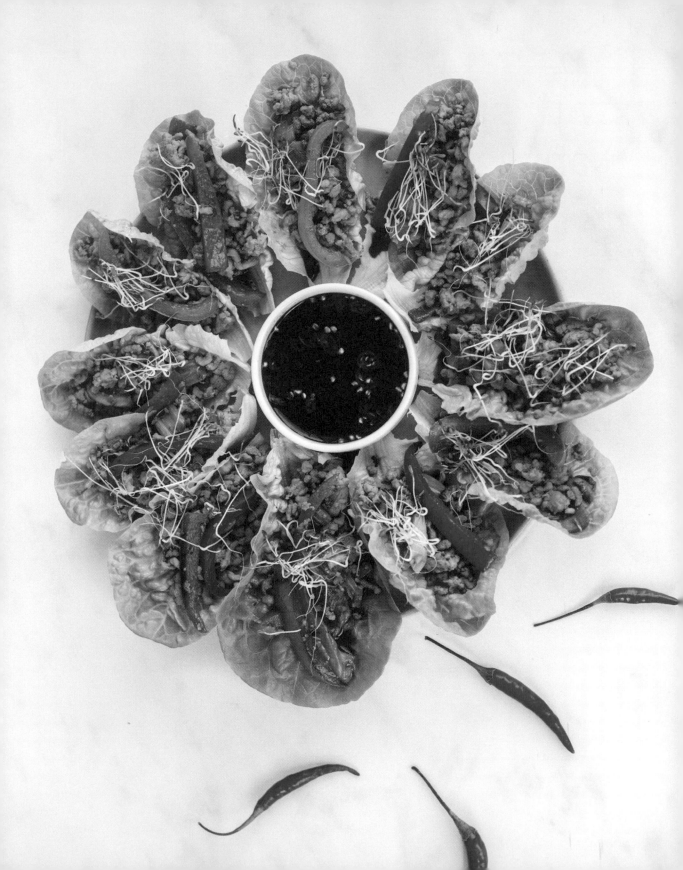

- baby gem or butterhead lettuce leaves (3-4 large leaves per portion)
- 1 tbsp toasted sesame oil
- 4 garlic cloves, crushed
- 1 fresh red chilli, deseeded and finely chopped
- 1 tsp ginger paste
- 480g minced pork
- 8 chestnut mushrooms, thinly sliced
- 2 large celery sticks, finely chopped
- 3 spring onions, thinly sliced
- 1 green pepper, thinly sliced
- 1 red pepper, thinly sliced
- 3 tbsp sugar-free soy sauce
- 1 tbsp fish sauce
- alfalfa, to garnish (optional)

**FOR THE SPICY CABBAGE:**
- 600g white cabbage, thinly shredded
- 2 tbsp coconut oil
- 4 garlic cloves, crushed
- 1 fresh red chilli, deseeded and finely chopped
- 3 tsp massaman curry paste

## HOW TO PREPARE

1 Prepare the lettuce leaves by gently separating the large leaves from the stem. You may need up to three heads of lettuce to get enough of the bigger outer leaves. Wash them and gently pat dry with kitchen paper. Set aside.

2 Heat the sesame oil in a wok or a large non-stick saucepan. Add the garlic, chilli and ginger paste and sauté on a low heat for 1 minute, until fragrant. Add the mince a bit at a time to brown in batches.

3 While the mince is browning, steam the cabbage for 10 minutes, until it's still crunchy.

4 Gradually add the mushrooms, celery, spring onions and peppers to the cooked mince until the vegetables are cooked to your liking. Season with the soy and fish sauces and keep warm.

5 Heat the coconut oil in a large non-stick pan. Add the garlic, chilli and curry paste and sauté for 1 minute, until fragrant. Add the steamed cabbage and stir well for even seasoning. Set aside, keeping it warm.

6 Spoon the hot mince into the lettuce cups and garnish each one with alfalfa (if using). Serve with the spicy cabbage on the side.

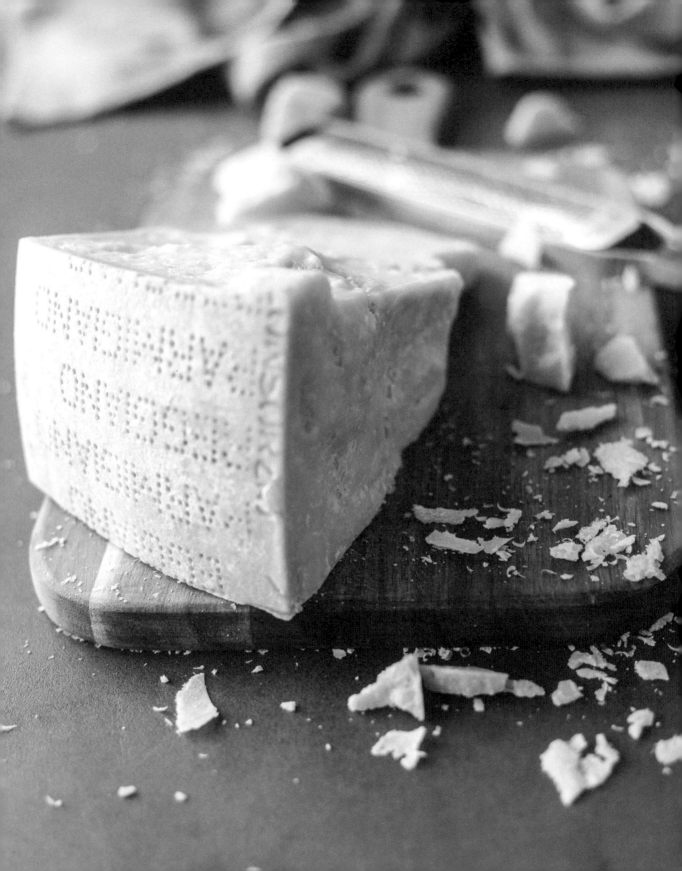

# Spaghetti carbonara

Having open packets of cheese in the fridge can be tempting, so grate the leftovers into a Ziplock bag and freeze for later. Be ready to eat this dish as soon as it's done, as it doesn't keep very well.

— 2 eggs
— 20g Parmesan cheese, grated
— 20g feta cheese, crumbled
— pinch of dried oregano
— freshly ground black pepper
— 2 bacon medallions, finely chopped
— 1 bag of Eurodiet Konjac spaghetti, rinsed well
— green salad or green vegetables, to serve

## HOW TO PREPARE

1 Mix the eggs, Parmesan and feta in a bowl. Season with a pinch of oregano and black pepper. Set aside.
2 Fry the bacon in a non-stick pan until cooked through, then add to the eggs along with the rinsed spaghetti. Mix everything through so that the sauce and spaghetti are hot.
3 Serve with a green salad or green vegetables on the side.

# Pasta Bolognese

Traditional white spaghetti has over 70g of carbohydrates per 100g, which is why I've used konjac spaghetti instead for this low-carbohydrate recipe. It contains no carbohydrates at all, but it makes you feel like you're having them, plus the fibre it contains makes you feel full. My patients love this recipe. They often say that it's all in the head when it comes to dieting, and if you don't feel deprived, you can stick to it!

— 1 tbsp olive oil
— 1 leek, washed and chopped
— 1 courgette, chopped
— 100g chestnut mushrooms, sliced
— 240g minced beef, pork or lamb
— 1 packet of Eurodiet konjac spaghetti, rinsed well
— 2 x 400g tins of whole peeled plum tomatoes
— ½ tsp paprika
— ½ beef stock cube
— freshly ground black pepper
— 20g Parmesan cheese, grated
— fresh basil, to garnish

## HOW TO PREPARE

1 Heat the oil in a large non-stick pan. Add the leek, courgette and mushrooms and sauté for 5 minutes, until soft. Add the mince and cook for 5 minutes more. Add the tomatoes and paprika and crumble in the beef stock cube. Cook for 25 minutes, stirring frequently.

2 Once the sauce is cooked, add the spaghetti and heat through, then season to taste with black pepper. Serve with the grated Parmesan on top and garnish with a sprig of fresh basil.

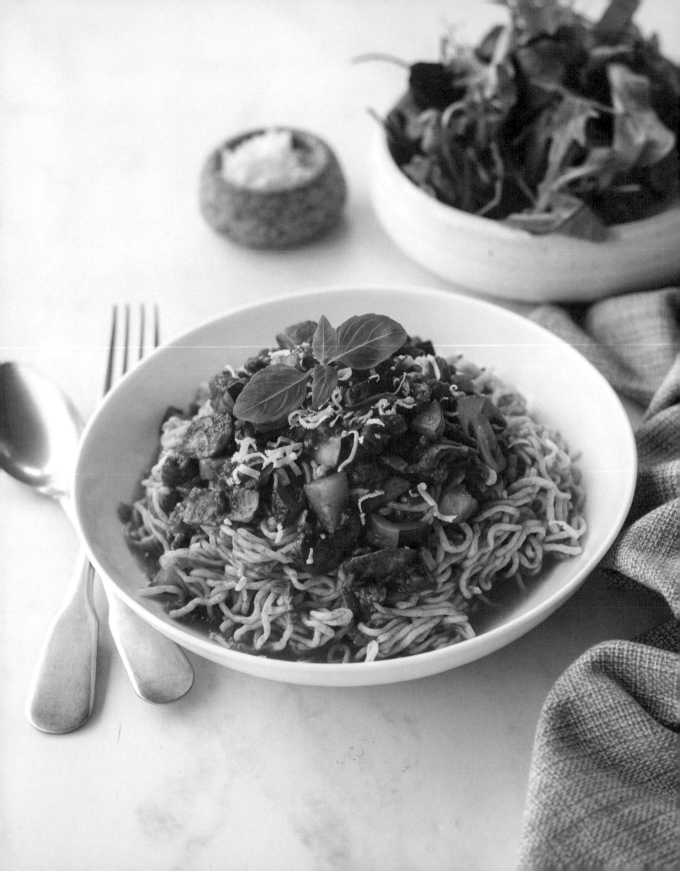

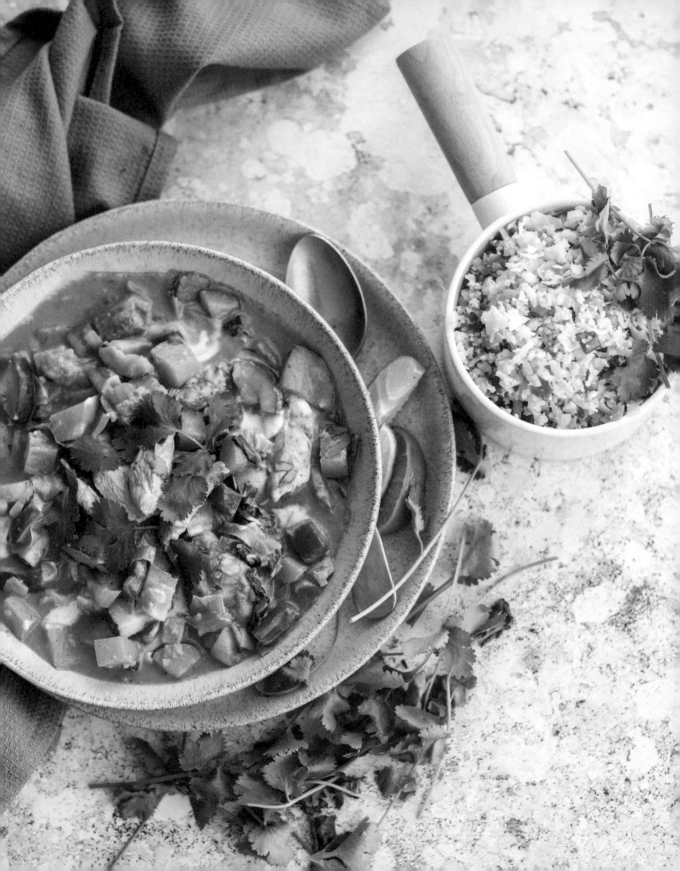

# Chicken and turnip curry

PHASE 2 ONWARDS | SERVES 2

In this recipe, the turnip (or swede) takes on a whole new twist. Turnip has only a fraction of the carbohydrates when compared to a potato, yet it can be used to take its place in many dishes.

— 300g turnip, peeled and cut into small cubes

— 1 tbsp coconut oil

— 1 tbsp Panang curry paste (red or yellow curry paste would also work)

— 1 leek, washed and chopped

— 2 garlic cloves, crushed

— 2 x 150g chicken fillets, cut into thin strips

— 1 courgette, chopped

— ½ red pepper, chopped

— 2 pak choi, chopped

— 4 kaffir lime leaves

— 120ml full-fat coconut milk

— 4 tbsp finely chopped fresh coriander, plus extra leaves to garnish

— 2 tsp soy sauce (make sure it's sugar-free)

— juice of 1 small lime

— cauliflower rice (page 196), to serve

— lime wedges, to serve

## HOW TO PREPARE

1 Place the turnip in a steamer. Steam for 10–15 minutes, until soft but not soggy.

2 Meanwhile, heat the coconut oil in a non-stick pan. Add the curry paste and mix together with the oil once the oil starts melting. Add the leek and garlic and sauté for 3 minutes. Add the chicken and cook for 5 minutes, then add the courgette and pepper and cook for a further 5 minutes, stirring frequently.

3 Add the steamed turnip along with the pak choi, kaffir lime leaves, coconut milk, coriander and soy sauce, then pour in the lime juice and 100ml of hot water from the kettle. Simmer for 3 minutes.

4 Remove the kaffir lime leaves and garnish with whole coriander leaves. Serve the curry with cauliflower rice on the side and lime wedges for squeezing over.

# Lamb and feta burgers

PHASE 2 ONWARDS | MAKES 8 BURGERS
(2 BURGERS PER PORTION)

HOW TO PREPARE

These burgers are so satisfying that you really won't miss the bun. Choosing more vegetables and fewer carbohydrates is a must in long-term weight management and glucose control. Did you know that each burger bun could set you back by over 200 calories and over 30g of carbohydrates? It may not sound like much, but when you add up the daily totals, it could end up being the straw that broke the camel's back.

— 1 large courgette, grated
— 380g lamb mince
— 60g feta cheese
— 1 bunch of spring onions, finely chopped
— 1 tbsp sugar-free soy sauce
— mixture of fresh mint, coriander and parsley leaves, chopped finely
— freshly ground black pepper
— 2 tsp butter

1  Squeeze the excess water from the grated courgette. Place all the ingredients except the butter in a mixing bowl, reserving some of the herbs for garnish. Mix well with your hands to combine, then form into eight burgers.
2  Melt the butter in a large chargrill pan set over a medium heat. Add the burgers and grill until cooked, turning halfway through.
3  Garnish the burgers with the remaining fresh herbs and serve with a vegetable side of your choice.

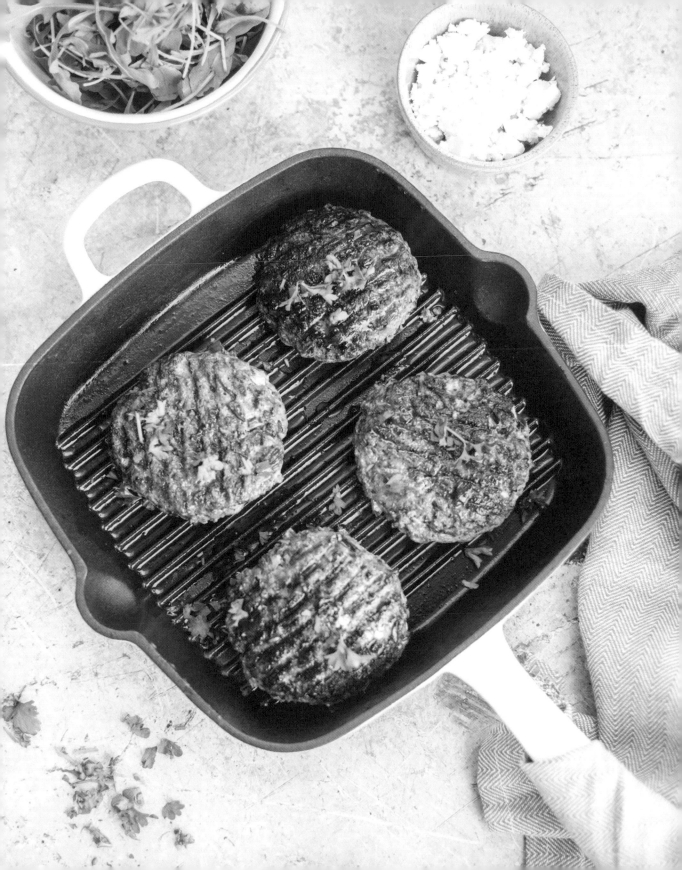

# Pork in black bean sauce

PHASE 2 ONWARDS | SERVES 2

This is for those of you who have been missing your Chinese take-away. You would honestly spend more time between the phone call and waiting for the delivery than making this dish yourself. This black bean and garlic sauce is so strong that you don't need any more than a tablespoon between two servings and it's available in most big supermarkets. Shiitake mushrooms are much meatier (and tastier) than the typical button mushrooms and can make a real difference in this dish. Look for a nice firm skin when buying them.

— 1 tsp coconut oil
— 1 tbsp Lee Kum Kee black bean garlic sauce
— 250g pork steak, cut into thin strips
— 1 yellow pepper, sliced
— 1 orange pepper, sliced
— 150g leek, washed and thinly sliced
— 100g shiitake mushrooms
— 200g bean sprouts
— 1 bag of Eurodiet konjac rice, rinsed well

HOW TO PREPAPRE

1 Heat the coconut oil and black bean sauce together in a non-stick pan. Add the pork and brown the meat, then add the peppers, leek and mushrooms. Cook until the pork and vegetables are cooked through.
2 Add the bean sprouts and cook for a further 2–3 minutes, then add the rinsed konjac rice and heat through. Serve hot.

# Prawns
# with konjac
# spaghetti

PHASE 2 ONWARDS | SERVES 1

HOW TO PREPARE

This is a quick but very tasty weeknight meal. Swap the prawns for chicken if you don't like them and try red curry paste instead of yellow.

— 1 tsp coconut oil
— ½ tsp yellow curry paste
— ½ orange pepper, sliced thinly
— 3 spring onions, finely chopped
— ½ tsp grated fresh ginger
— 1 pak choi, chopped
— 200g cooked prawns
— 1 bag of Eurodiet konjac spaghetti, rinsed well
— 10 drops of Biona hot pepper sauce (or to taste)
— 1 tsp brown rice vinegar
— ½ tsp fish sauce
— dash of sugar-free soy sauce
— squeeze of lime juice
— fresh coriander, to garnish

1   Heat the coconut oil and curry paste together in a non-stick pan. Add the pepper, spring onions and ginger and sauté for 2–3 minutes. Add the pak choi, prawns and spaghetti and heat through.
2   Season with the hot pepper sauce, brown rice vinegar, fish sauce, soy sauce and lime juice. Stir through the chopped fresh coriander just before serving.

# Jambalaya

Chorizo sausage has an amazing flavour and it is well worth paying a little extra for a good-quality one. It has a lot of calories, though, so use it sparingly. There are as many variations of this Louisiana dish as there are people who love it, so feel free to vary the contents to suit your taste buds. You could swap the prawns and chorizo for pork sausage and chicken, for example. Once you have finished with the initial phases of the diet, you can swap the spring onions for regular onions and try some brown rice instead of the konjac rice.

— 1 tsp butter
— 60g dry-cured chorizo, peeled if necessary and cut into small cubes
— 1 green pepper, finely chopped
— 1 yellow pepper, finely chopped
— 1 bunch of spring onions, chopped
— 2 garlic cloves, crushed
— 400g tin of cherry tomatoes
— 1 tbsp Biona hot pepper sauce or Tabasco sauce
— 1 tsp ground turmeric
— pinch of Cajun seasoning (optional)
— 150g cooked king prawns
— 1 bag of Eurodiet konjac rice, rinsed well
— 1 fresh red chilli, deseeded and finely chopped (optional)
— fresh coriander or parsley, to garnish (optional)
— lime wedges, to serve

## HOW TO PREPAPRE

1 Melt the butter in a non-stick frying pan, then add the chorizo pieces and fry until they are a little crispy. Add the peppers, spring onions and garlic and fry for a further 3 minutes, stirring occasionally.

2 Pour in the tinned cherry tomatoes and add the hot pepper sauce and turmeric. Check for seasoning, adding more hot pepper sauce or a pinch of Cajun seasoning (if using). Add the cooked prawns and the rinsed konjac rice and heat through. Garnish with the chilli and fresh coriander or parsley (if using) and serve hot with lime wedges on the side for squeezing over.

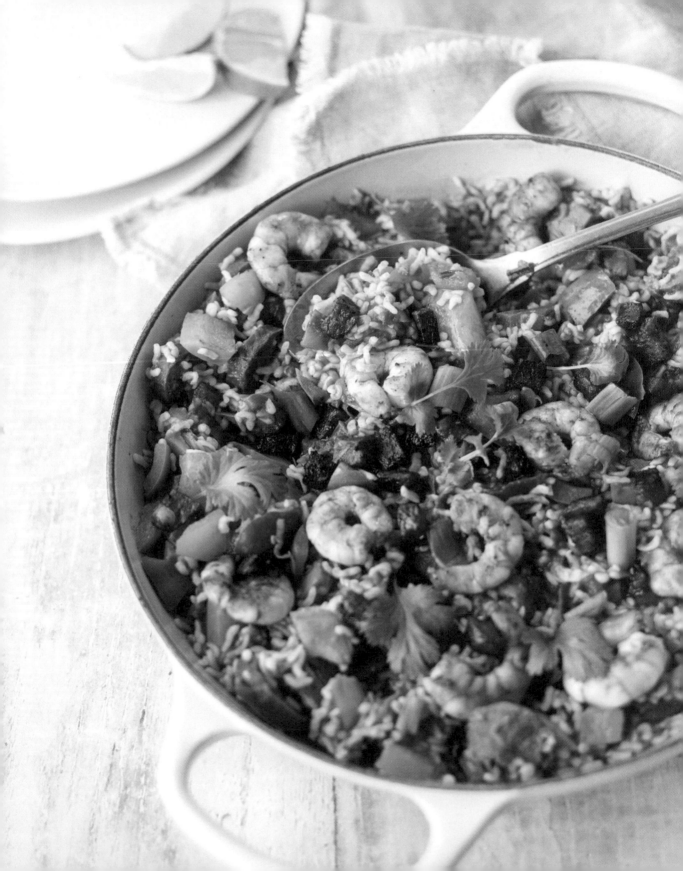

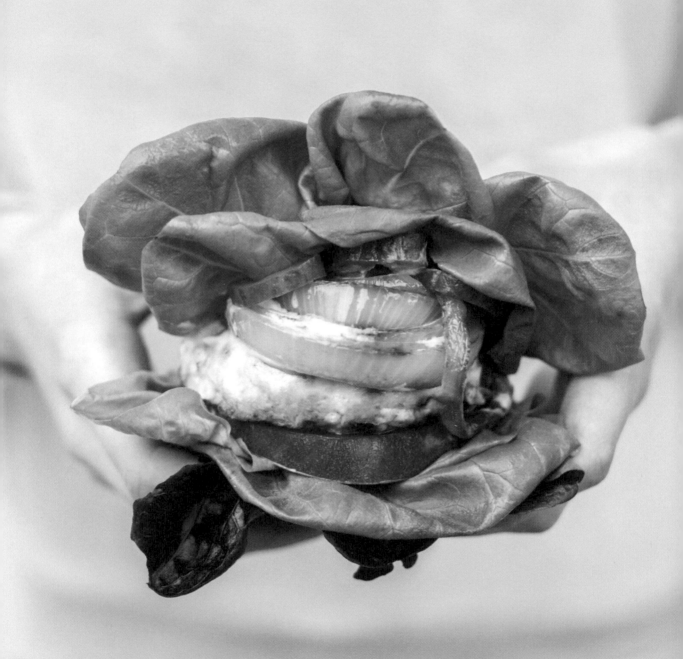

# Turkey and horseradish burgers

These burgers are so quick to make that you could make two batches at the same time and freeze the extras for a simple weeknight dinner. They are low in calories and carbohydrates. Some horseradish sauces are hotter than others, so test the one you have before adding the full amount.

— **600g turkey mince**
— **3-4 tbsp horseradish sauce**
— **1 tsp Herbamare salt**
— **1 tbsp butter**
— **iceberg or butterhead lettuce leaves**
— **sliced tomatoes, to serve**
— **sliced large gherkins, to serve**

## HOW TO PREPARE

1 Mix the turkey mince with the horseradish sauce and Herbamare salt using your hands. Form into four large burgers.
2 Melt the butter in a large non-stick frying pan. Add the burgers to the pan and cook on a medium heat for 15–20 minutes, until fully cooked through, turning frequently.
3 Serve in between large lettuce leaves instead of a bun with tomato slices, gherkins and any optional extras and your side of choice.

# Chicken and aubergine bake

PHASE 2 ONWARDS | SERVES 2

The only complaint I've ever had about this dish is that the portion can be too big to finish! The beauty of being in ketosis is that you really don't feel hungry. Try using beef or chicken mince for this recipe or replace the aubergine layers with thinly shaved slices of courgettes. Double up the serving and freeze it in portions for a quick weekday meal.

— **3 medium aubergines, peeled and sliced very thinly**
— **Herbamare salt**
— **3 tbsp olive oil**
— **5 garlic cloves, crushed**
— **300g chicken fillets, thinly sliced**
— **5 mushrooms, thinly sliced**
— **½ a courgette, finely chopped**
— **500ml tomato passata**
— **2 tbsp tomato purée**
— **1 tbsp Biona hot pepper sauce**
— **20g Parmesan cheese, grated**

## HOW TO PREPARE

1 Salt both sides of the aubergine slices with the Herbamare salt. Place the slices in a colander set in the sink for 20 minutes to draw out the excess water.

2 Preheat the oven to 180°C.

3 Once they're ready, rinse the salt off the aubergines and gently pat them dry using kitchen paper. Place the slices on a non-stick baking tray. Brush them with 2 tablespoons of the olive oil using a pastry brush. Cook in the oven for 10 minutes.

4 Meanwhile, to make the chicken sauce, heat the remaining tablespoon of oil in a non-stick saucepan. Add the garlic and sauté for 1 minute, until fragrant. Add the chicken, mushrooms, courgette, passata, tomato purée and hot pepper sauce and cook for 5 minutes.

5 Remove the aubergines from the oven. Place one layer of slices on the bottom of a 15cm x 30cm baking dish. Add a layer of sauce, then cover with another layer of aubergines. Top with another layer of sauce and finish with a layer of aubergines.

6 Bake in the centre of the oven for 20 minutes. Sprinkle the Parmesan on top just before removing from the oven to allow it to melt.

# Chilli sin carne

Chilli and rice go hand in hand, so try this vegetarian version or serve with cauliflower rice or konjac rice from Phase 3 onwards, or with some brown rice or sour cream during your maintenance phase. Tinned beans are incredibly handy and you can easily make large batches of food with them with minimal effort. They're also a good source of protein and fibre.

— 1 tbsp olive oil
— 4 carrots, peeled and finely chopped
— 2 red onions, chopped
— 5 garlic cloves, crushed
— 1 green pepper, chopped
— 1 red pepper, chopped
— 400g tin of red kidney beans, drained and rinsed
— 400g tin of black beans, drained and rinsed
— 200g ready-made fresh salsa
— 1 tbsp Worcester sauce
— 1–2 tsp cayenne pepper (depending on how hot you like it)
— 1 tsp ground cumin
— vegetable bouillon (optional)
— chopped fresh coriander, to garnish

## HOW TO PREPARE

1 Heat the oil in a large, deep non-stick pan. Add the carrots, onion and garlic and sauté for 5 minutes. Add the peppers and cook for another 5 minutes, stirring. Add the beans, salsa, Worcester sauce, cayenne and cumin. Cook on a low heat for another 3 minutes to heat the beans through.

2 Taste for seasoning and add a little vegetable bouillon if desired. Garnish with chopped fresh coriander and serve with a side of your choice (see the introduction for suggestions).

# Fiery pizza with spicy pepperoni and jalapeño peppers

Making the pizza base from scratch leaves you in charge of what goes in it. You may have only made the base with regular white flour before this, but try swapping it for wholemeal spelt flour, as it has a superior fibre content and nutritional value. Thankfully you can now buy it from large supermarkets and health food stores.

- 1 x 7g sachet of fast-action yeast
- ½ tsp sea salt
- 150ml lukewarm water
- 1 tbsp olive oil
- 300g wholemeal spelt flour, plus extra for dusting
- handful of rocket leaves, to serve

**FOR THE TOPPINGS:**
- 400g tin of pizza sauce (Mutti brand is my favourite)
- a few drops of Biona hot pepper sauce or Tabasco sauce
- 200g pepperoni
- jalapeño slices from a jar, drained and patted dry (to taste)
- 200g grated mozzarella cheese

## HOW TO PREPARE

1 Put the yeast and salt into a mixing bowl, then add the lukewarm water and oil. Start adding the flour and mix to create a dough. Form the dough into a ball, then place it back in the bowl and cover with a clean tea towel. Leave to rise in a warm place for approximately 1 hour.

2 Preheat the oven to 200°C. Line a baking tray with non-stick baking paper.

3 Dust a small amount of flour on a clean work surface. Tip the dough out onto it and use your fingers or a rolling pin to shape it into a round base. Use the rolling pin to lift the base onto the lined baking tray.

4 Spread the pizza sauce over the base and sprinkle evenly with the hot pepper sauce. Spread the pepperoni and jalapeño slices evenly over the base and top with the grated cheese.

5 Cook in the centre of the oven for 12 minutes. Serve with the rocket as a side salad.

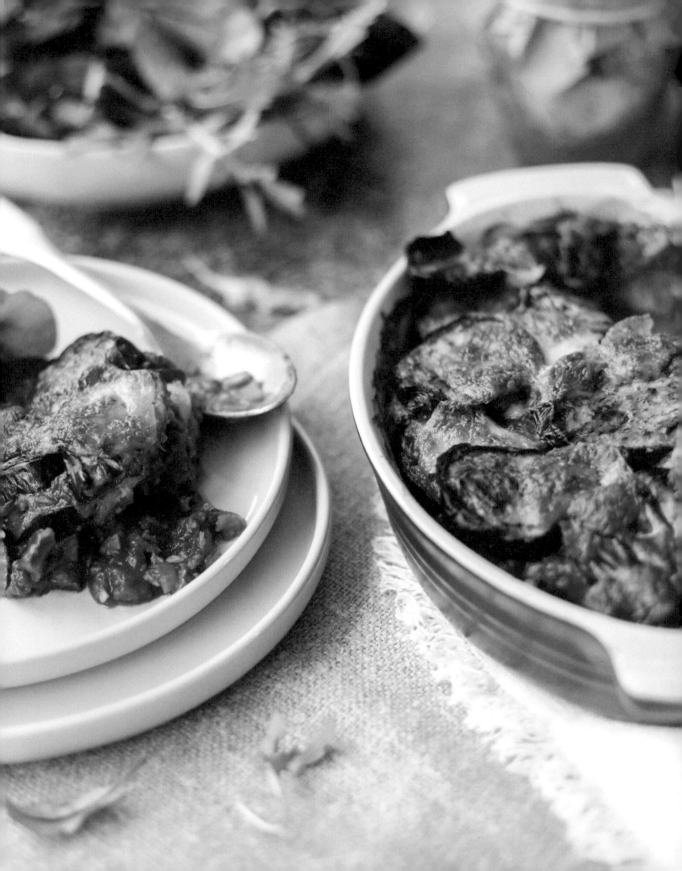

# Moussaka

MAINTENANCE | SERVES 4

HOW TO PREPARE

This moussaka is very satisfying without the creamy béchamel sauce that many chefs use in their recipes. I've further reduced the calorie load by grilling the aubergines instead of frying them. You can make your moussaka slightly different each time by changing the seasonings or the choice of meat. Try it with bay leaves and oregano, or simmer the sauce for a little longer with a cinnamon stick and a splash of red wine.

— 1 beef stock cube
— 4 aubergines
— salt and freshly ground black pepper
— 1 tbsp olive oil
— 4 onions, sliced
— 4 garlic cloves, crushed
— 480g lean minced beef or lamb
— 4 courgettes, finely chopped
— 4 x 400g tins of chopped tomatoes
— spray oil
— 4 small sweet potatoes, peeled and sliced
— 200g mozzarella cheese, thinly sliced
— 100g strong Cheddar cheese, grated

1 Dissolve the beef stock cube in 200ml of boiling water.
2 Cut the aubergines into thin round slices. Place on a dish side by side and sprinkle with salt. Leave to sweat for a minimum of 20 minutes to draw out the excess water.
3 Meanwhile, heat the oil in a large pan. Add the onions and garlic and sauté until soft, then add the meat and fry for a few minutes. Stir in the courgettes, chopped tomatoes and beef stock. Leave to simmer without a lid to evaporate the excess water, stirring occasionally.
4 Preheat the grill.
5 Rinse the salt off the aubergine slices and pat them dry with kitchen paper. Lightly spray a large baking tray with spray oil and place the aubergine slices on it. Place under the grill for 10 minutes.
6 Spray a large, deep ovenproof dish with spray oil, then place the sweet potato slices on the bottom of the dish. Pour the meat sauce over the sweet potato, then place the grilled aubergine slices on top. Finish with a layer of the thinly sliced mozzarella.
7 Cover the dish with tin foil and cook the moussaka in the oven for 45 minutes, adding the grated Cheddar cheese 10 minutes before the end of the cooking time.

# Vegetarian burgers with tzatziki and quinoa

MAINTENANCE | SERVES 4

I've lost count of the number of patients who think quinoa is just protein, the same as, say, chicken. Yes, it is a source of protein, as it has all nine essential amino acids, but it still consists primarily of carbohydrates. The food industry has gone mad trying to put it in products such as wraps and breads – I've even seen it in yoghurt. Most of the time the portion of quinoa in the product is minimal, as quinoa is not a cheap ingredient. If you want to introduce it to your diet, it can be introduced from Phase 3 onwards. It can replace couscous in many recipes as a more nutritious carbohydrate.

- 1 vegetable stock cube
- 1kg butternut squash, peeled and finely chopped
- 3 high-fibre slim rye crispbreads (the Finn Crisp brand work best)
- 400g tin of chickpeas, drained and rinsed
- 1 tsp Herbamare salt
- 1 small egg, lightly beaten

**FOR THE TZATZIKI:**
- 200ml natural yoghurt
- 1 cucumber (approximately 350g), grated after seeds are removed
- 3 garlic cloves, crushed
- 10 fresh mint leaves, chopped
- pinch of salt

**TO SERVE:**
- 200g quinoa

1. Put the vegetable stock cube in a large saucepan with 1 litre of water and bring to the boil, stirring to dissolve the stock cube. Add the squash and simmer for about 10 minutes, until soft.
2. While the butternut squash is cooking, put the rye crispbreads into a ziplock bag and crush them with a rolling pin.
3. Prepare the tzatziki by mixing all the ingredients together in a bowl. Store in the fridge until ready to use.
4. Drain the cooked butternut squash and place the cubes on a large tray to cool down.
5. Preheat the oven to 200°C. Line a large baking tray with non-stick baking paper.
6. Mix the cooled butternut squash with the crispbread crumbs, drained chickpeas and Herbamare salt. Mash well to combine. Add the egg and mix through.
7. Using a tablespoon, make small burger patties and place them side by side on the lined baking tray. Bake in the oven for 12–15 minutes, until slightly golden.
8. Meanwhile, prepare the quinoa according to the packet instructions.
9. Remove the burgers from the oven and serve with the quinoa and tzatziki on the side.

# Fish cakes

I like my fish cakes baked rather than
fried. They won't get as 'crumby', but
I like to taste the fish rather than fried
breadcrumbs. You can make this dish
very quickly from leftover mashed
potatoes. If you are afraid of fish bones,
ask the fishmonger to give you the tail
ends of the fish, as these contain fewer
bones. Smoked coley gives a wonderful
flavour to this comfort food.

— 500g potatoes, peeled and sliced
— 300g fresh boneless white fish, such as hake
— 150g boneless smoked coley
— 2 tbsp low-fat crème fraîche
— 2 tbsp sugar-free soy sauce
— 1 tbsp chopped fresh flat-leaf parsley
— 1 tbsp chopped fresh coriander
— pinch of dried herbs, such as dill or parsley
  (optional)
— ground almonds, for dusting
— 60ml sweet chilli sauce, to serve (optional)
— ½ a fresh red chilli, deseeded and thinly sliced
  (optional)
— lemon wedges, to serve

## HOW TO PREPARE

1  Place the sliced potatoes in a saucepan.
   Cover with water and bring to the boil.
   Reduce the heat and cook until they
   are soft enough for mashing. Drain and
   transfer to a large bowl, then mash until
   smooth. Set aside to cool.

2  Bring some water to the boil in a double
   boiler. Place the white fish and smoked
   coley in the steaming insert and steam
   for 10 minutes.

3  Preheat the oven to 200°C. Line a large
   baking tray with non-stick baking paper.

4  Once the mashed potatoes have cooled,
   stir in the cooked fish and crème
   fraîche, then add the soy sauce and
   chopped fresh herbs and mix well. Taste
   for seasoning and adjust as desired,
   adding more soy sauce or a pinch of
   dried herbs (if using).

5  Shape the mixture into 12 cakes. Lightly
   dust each one with ground almonds and
   place on the lined tray.

6  Place the tray on the top shelf of the
   oven and bake for 10–15 minutes, until
   the fish cakes are lightly browned.
   Serve with a small dish of sweet chilli
   sauce with a few slices of fresh red chilli
   added to it (if using), lemon wedges and
   vegetables of your choice.

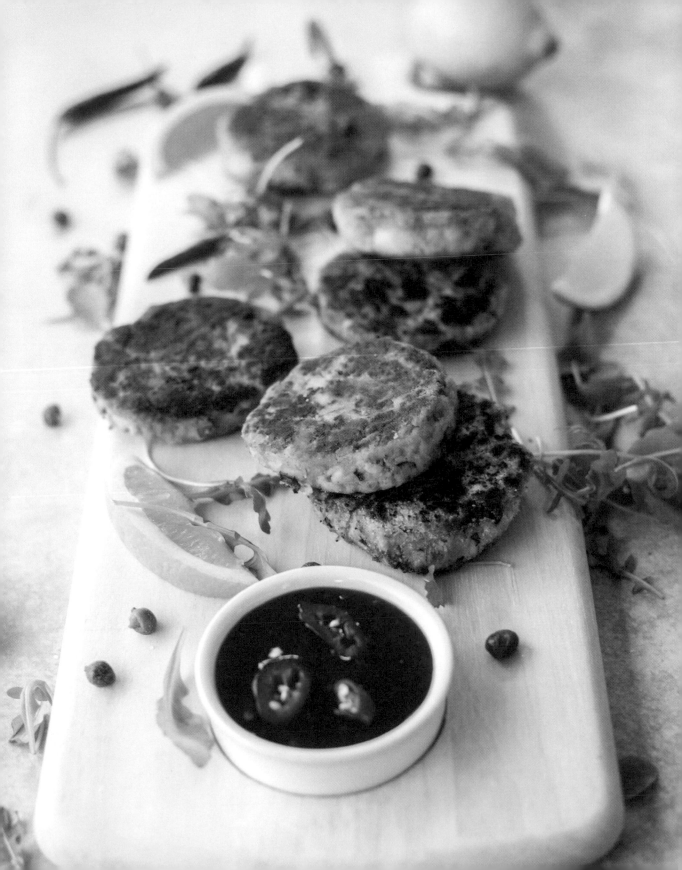

# Cape Malay-style fish curry

MAINTENANCE | SERVES 4

I lived in South Africa before moving to Ireland. The local cuisine offers a huge mixture of different flavours. There are many different ways to make a Cape Malay curry, but I've tried to limit the sugar and carbohydrate content in my version. If you are doing well and your HbA1c has remained stable, you could add a little mango chutney to this sauce to give it some sweetness.

— 1 tbsp olive oil
— 3 onions, chopped
— 5 garlic cloves, crushed
— 5 cardamom pods, seeds ground with a pestle and mortar
— 1 tsp garam masala
— 1 tsp ground turmeric
— 1 tsp ground coriander
— 1 tsp ground cumin
— 1 tsp ground cinnamon
— 4 medium potatoes or sweet potatoes, cut into small cubes
— 1 x 400g tin of whole peeled plum tomatoes
— 800g firm white fish, such as monkfish
— 450g frozen peas, defrosted with boiled water
— 2 tbsp sugar-free soy sauce
— chopped fresh coriander, to garnish (optional)

HOW TO PREPARE

1 Heat the oil in a large non-stick pan. Add the onions, garlic and all the spices. Fry gently for 2 minutes to release their aromas.
2 Add the potatoes and tinned tomatoes. Cover with a lid and cook for 10–15 minutes. Add a little boiling water if needed.
3 Add the fish, thawed peas and soy sauce. Cover with the lid again and cook for 5 minutes, until the fish is cooked. Garnish with chopped fresh coriander (if using).

# Beef and red wine casserole

Casseroles are so handy and work well with a number of different ingredients – you can swap most of the ingredients in this dish to suit your preferences. It is very important that your maintenance phase is not putting you under pressure, but that you are enjoying the newly introduced foods and that you keep trying new healthy foods. Gherkins can really make this casserole unlike any you have tried before.

— 1 beef stock cube
— 1 tbsp butter
— 480g sirloin steak, thinly sliced
— 5 slices of bacon, finely chopped
— 2 onions, sliced
— 4 garlic cloves, crushed
— 2 large sweet potatoes, cut into chunks
— 2 celery sticks, chopped
— 200g mushrooms, cut into quarters
— 2 x 400g tins of whole peeled plum tomatoes
— 6 sprigs of fresh thyme
— 5 bay leaves
— 200g large gherkins, finely chopped
— 250ml red wine
— Herbamare salt
— freshly ground black pepper

## HOW TO PREPARE

1. Dissolve the beef stock cube in 200ml of boiling water.
2. Melt the butter in a wok or large, deep pan. Add the beef and bacon and stir continuously to avoid them sticking to the pan. Once the beef is browned, add the onions and garlic and reduce the heat. You may need to add a little of the stock at this stage.
3. Add the sweet potatoes, celery, mushrooms, tinned tomatoes, stock, thyme sprigs and bay leaves. Cover with a lid and simmer for 15–20 minutes, until the potatoes are almost cooked. Add more stock if required.
4. Add the gherkins and red wine and taste for seasoning. Add Herbamare salt if required and some freshly ground black pepper. Simmer for a further 3 minutes. Remove the thyme sprigs and bay leaves before serving.

# Hunter's casserole

This casserole is a great example of how you can reintroduce all the foods you may have been missing during the early stages of the plan. Guinness gives the stock a beautiful taste and richness, yet the alcohol will simmer away during the long cooking. Alcohol can't be consumed at the start of your diet because it can stop the ketosis and delay your weight loss. Stick this casserole in the oven on a bright Sunday afternoon, get your walking shoes on and come home to a satisfying hot meal.

— **1 beef stock cube**
— **2 tsp butter**
— **4 venison sausages**
— **260g black pudding, cut into thick slices**
— **10 carrots, peeled and chopped**
— **6 pickled onions**
— **4 celery sticks, chopped**
— **4 garlic cloves, crushed**
— **10 sprigs of fresh thyme**
— **2 sprigs of fresh rosemary**
— **500ml Guinness**
— **fresh thyme, to garnish**

## HOW TO PREPARE

1 Dissolve the beef stock cube in 500ml of boiling water.
2 Preheat the oven to 180°C.
3 Heat the butter in a large non-stick pan. Add the sausages and brown them in the butter. Add the black pudding and fry on both sides.
4 Place all the vegetables, garlic and herbs in a large, deep casserole. Pour in the Guinness and stock. Slice the sausages, then add to the casserole along with the black pudding.
5 Cover with the lid, then place the casserole in the oven and cook for 60 minutes. Reduce the heat to 160°C and cook for a further 30 minutes. Garnish with fresh thyme.

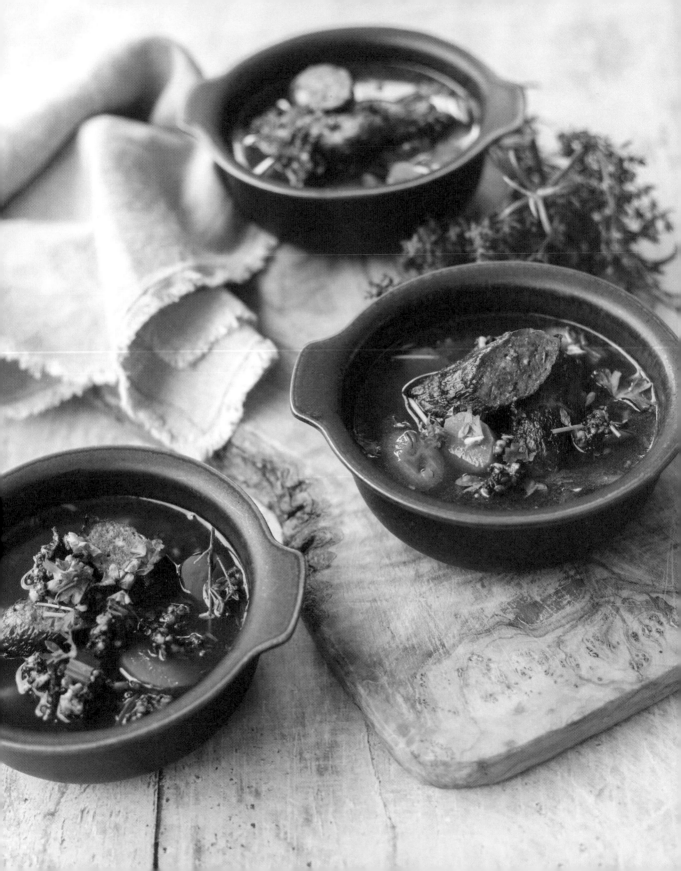

# Vegetarian lasagne

Did you know that vegetables contain some protein? Spinach has almost 3g of protein per 100g, so each serving of this lasagne already has over 5g of protein just from the spinach! I hope you enjoy my meat-free version of a lasagne.

— 1 tbsp olive oil
— 1 onion, chopped
— 2 garlic cloves, crushed
— 2 x 400g tins of chopped tomatoes
— 1 tbsp vegetable bouillon
— 750g spinach, washed
— 1 tbsp tomato purée
— 1 tsp dried oregano
— pinch of paprika
— freshly ground black pepper
— spray oil
— 10 whole wheat lasagne sheets
— 150g grated mozzarella cheese

FOR THE WHITE SAUCE:
— 20g butter
— 3 tbsp plain flour
— 800ml milk

## HOW TO PREPARE

1 Heat the oil in a large non-stick pan. Add the onion and garlic and fry for a few minutes. Add the chopped tomatoes, vegetable bouillon and half of the spinach. Cover and let the spinach wilt into the sauce. Stir the sauce, then add the rest of the spinach.

2 Stir in the tomato purée, oregano, paprika and black pepper. Let it simmer for 3 minutes, stirring occasionally. Remove from the heat and set aside.

3 To make the white sauce, melt the butter in a non-stick pan. Add the flour and the milk, stirring continuously. The sauce is ready once it has become thick.

4 Preheat the oven to 200°C.

5 Use spray oil to coat a large rectangular baking dish. Spread a portion of the tomato sauce in the bottom of the dish, followed by a layer of lasagne sheets, then a layer of white sauce. Repeat these layers until all the sauce and lasagne sheets have been used up, finishing with a layer of white sauce.

6 Sprinkle the mozzarella cheese over the top. Cover the dish with tin foil and bake in the centre of the oven for 40 minutes, until cooked through.

# Yellow peppers stuffed with feta and pine nuts

Peppadews and feta cheese go nicely together in this maintenance dish. Peppadews are sold in jars and you can get either mild or hot varieties. Nuts in general have a very low carbohydrate content, but they can make weight loss difficult due to their high calorie content. Pine nuts are no exception: they contain almost 700 calories in just 100g!

— **200g brown rice**
— **8 yellow peppers**
— **1 tbsp olive oil**
— **1 large onion, chopped**
— **400g tin of chopped tomatoes**
— **50g peppadews, chopped**
— **1 tbsp tomato purée**
— **200g feta cheese, mashed with a fork**
— **100g pine nuts**

HOW TO PREPARE

2  Preheat the oven to 180°C.
3  Cook the brown rice according to the packet instructions. Once cooked, drain well.
4  Slice the tops off the peppers and set aside for later. Scrape out and discard all the seeds and white pith inside. Set them upright in an ovenproof dish.
5  While the rice is cooking, heat the olive oil in a large non-stick pan. Add the onion and sauté for a few minutes. Add the tinned tomatoes, peppadews and tomato purée and simmer for 10 minutes, uncovered.
6  Mix the cooked rice, tomato sauce, feta cheese and pine nuts together in a bowl. Fill the peppers with the rice mixture, then put the pepper lids back on top of the peppers.
7  Bake in the oven for 30 minutes, until the skin of the peppers starts to wrinkle and blister.

# Chicken fajitas

Most supermarkets now stock a variety of wraps, but many of them are made from white flour. Check the ingredients and choose one with only wholemeal wheat flour. This simple yoghurt-based take on the more traditional sour cream gives you all the flavour with half the calories, but not with any more sugars.

— 200g natural Greek yoghurt
— 1 garlic clove, crushed
— 1 tsp Herbamare salt
— 2 tsp butter
— 4 chicken fillets, cut in half lengthways
— 2 peppers, sliced lengthways
— 1 onion, sliced (or 1 bunch of spring onions, chopped)
— 4 big wholemeal wraps, or 8 small wraps
— 200g ready-made fresh salsa
— 200g strong Cheddar cheese, grated
— 1 bag of washed iceberg lettuce, shredded
— dash of sugar-free soy sauce
— guacamole (optional)
— finely chopped fresh coriander (optional)
— lime wedges, to serve

## HOW TO PREPARE

1 Mix the yoghurt with the crushed garlic and Herbamare salt. Cover and set aside in the fridge until ready to use.
2 Melt 1 teaspoon of the butter in a non-stick pan. Add the chicken and fry until cooked through, then remove from the pan. Cook the peppers and onion in the same pan until crisp. Keep warm.
3 Heat the remaining teaspoon of butter in a chargrill pan. Press the cooked chicken fillets on it to give them charred lines on both sides.
4 Add the tortilla wraps to the hot chargrill pan for a few seconds just to warm them up, taking care not to burn them.
5 Assemble the cooked chicken and vegetables in the middle of the wraps. Add the yoghurt dip, salsa, grated cheese, lettuce and soy sauce. Spoon in some guacamole and sprinkle with chopped fresh coriander (if using). Tightly roll up each wrap to close. Serve with a large side dish of vegetables or salad and lime wedges.

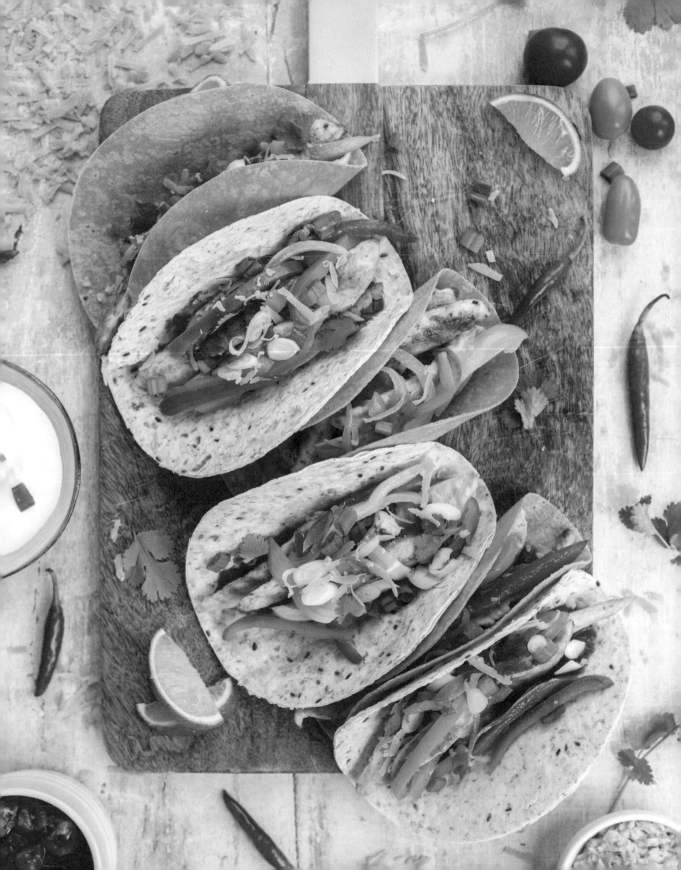

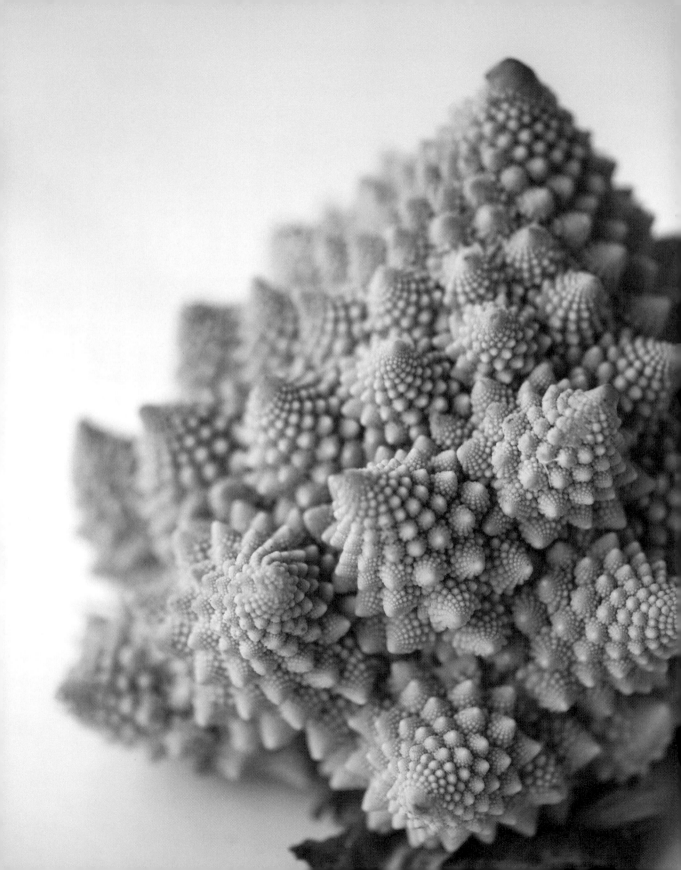

# CARBOHYDRATE SUBSTITUTES

# Cauliflower rice

Cauliflower rice has by now made it to the table of many low-carbohydrate dieters. Some supermarkets now stock it in their freezers, fresh vegetable sections or in vacuum-sealed bags. Although these may all come in handy at times, try my version with one of your main courses. Freshly grated cauliflower will always taste better.

— ½ tsp vegetable bouillon
— 1 tbsp oil
— ½ leek, washed and chopped
— 2 tsp dried parsley
— 1 tsp dried garlic
— ½ tsp chilli flakes
— 1 cauliflower, leaves removed and grated
— 2 spring onions, chopped

## HOW TO PREPARE

1 Dissolve the vegetable bouillon in 100ml of boiling water.
2 Heat the oil in a large non-stick frying pan. Add the leek and the dried parsley, garlic and chilli flakes. Fry for few minutes, then add the cauliflower and stock. Cover with a lid and cook on a low heat, stirring frequently. Once the 'rice' is cooked to your liking, stir in the spring onions. Serve as a side dish.

# Vegetable gratin

You really don't miss potatoes when you have great substitutes like this. One of the ways to not feel deprived is to make your plate look similar to what it used to look like. Although you can have only a heap of broccoli as your dinner vegetable portion, it's hardly going to be as satisfying as something like this. Make this dish to last you for a few nights or take a serving of it for your lunch instead of soup.

— 1 medium celeriac, peeled and chopped
— 1 medium cauliflower, cut into florets
— 1 medium head of broccoli, cut into florets
— 2 tbsp light cream cheese, plain or flavoured
— sea salt and freshly ground black pepper
— 10g Parmesan cheese shavings

## HOW TO PREPARE

1 Preheat the grill.
2 Place the chopped celeriac in a large saucepan. Cover with cold water, then cover the pan with a lid and bring to the boil. Boil the celeriac for 10–12 minutes.
3 Remove from the heat and add the cauliflower and broccoli to the same pan with their stems facing down. Replace the lid, bring back to the boil and cook for another 5 minutes, then drain well.
4 Mash all the vegetables together with the light cream cheese, then season to taste with salt and pepper.
5 Place in an ovenproof dish. Top with the Parmesan cheese shavings and place under the hot grill to brown. Serve with your main course.

# Mushroom risotto with konjac rice

Mushrooms are so versatile and incredibly low in both calories and carbohydrates. Mushroom foraging is very common in Finland and many families do it together. It's a great way to spend more time outdoors and breathe in the fresh forest air. I've used a beautiful selection of wild mushrooms for the photo, but any mushrooms will work just as well. Feel free to add more flavour to your risotto with garlic, or use flavoured soft cheese.

— 1 tsp butter
— 150g mushrooms, finely chopped
— 3 spring onions, finely chopped
— 1 bag of Eurodiet slim rice, rinsed
— 30g Philadelphia Light soft cheese
— 1 tbsp Worcester sauce
— ½ tsp vegetable bouillon
— freshly ground black pepper
— fresh flat-leaf parsley, finely chopped (optional)

## HOW TO PREPARE

1 Heat the butter in a non-stick pan. Add the mushrooms and spring onions and sauté for a few minutes, then add the rinsed Eurodiet slim rice and heat through. Add the soft cheese and mix well.
2 Season with the Worcester sauce, bouillon and some freshly ground black pepper. Garnish with the parsley (if using) and serve warm as a side to your main meal.

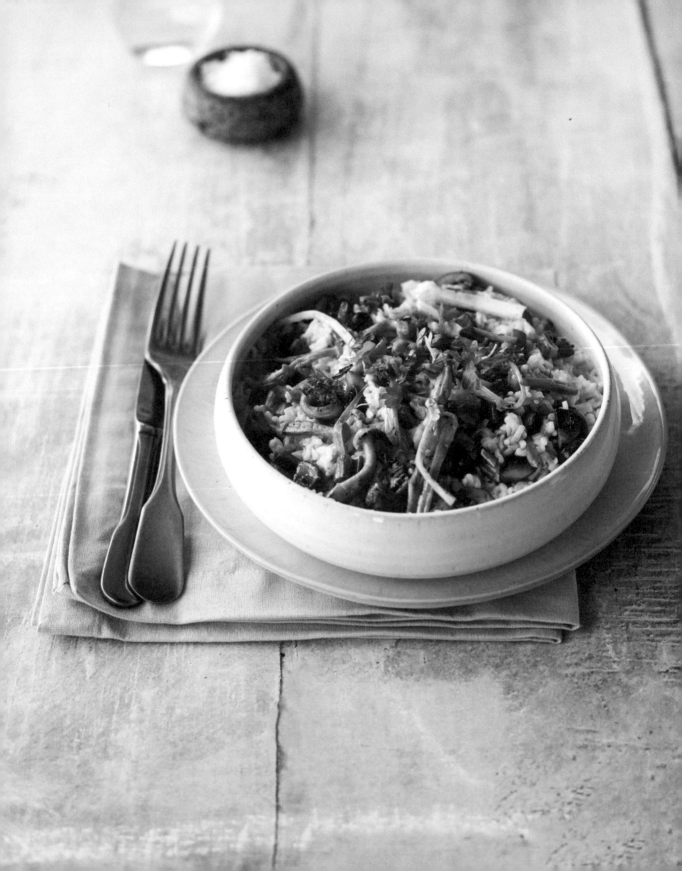

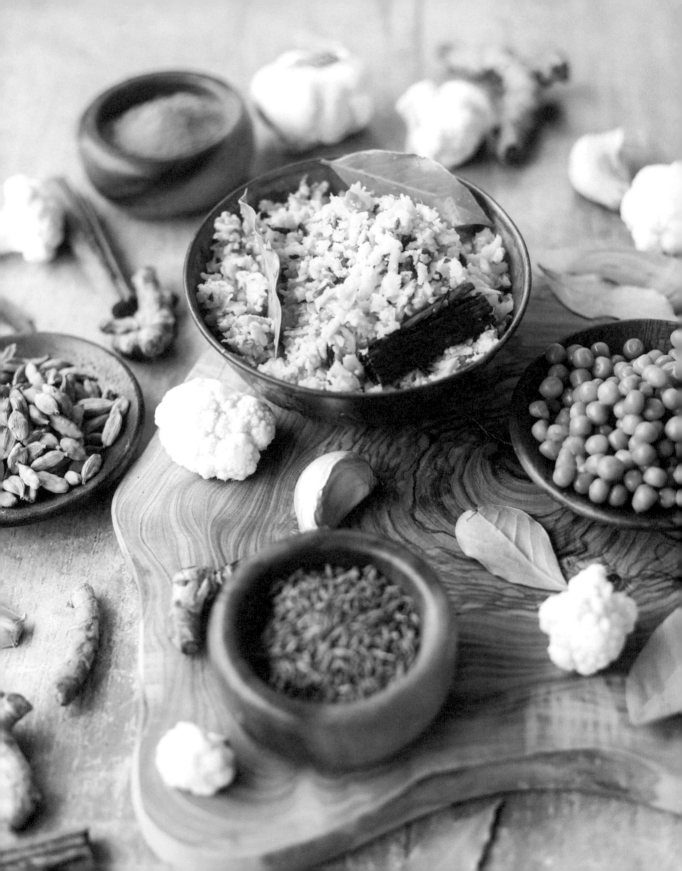

# Pilau cauliflower rice

It really takes no time to grate a head of cauliflower for this dish, but you can also use the frozen cauliflower 'rice' that is now sold in most supermarkets. You can add peas to your list of vegetables and into this side dish once you've finished with the ketogenic part of the diet.

— 1 tbsp butter
— 1 bunch of spring onions, chopped
— 2 garlic cloves, crushed
— 1 tsp cumin seeds
— 1 tsp ground turmeric
— 1 tsp sea salt
— 4 cardamom pods, bashed
— 2 bay leaves
— ½ cinnamon stick
— 1 large cauliflower, leaves removed and grated

## HOW TO PREPARE

1 Melt the butter in a non-stick pan. Add the spring onions, garlic, cumin seeds, turmeric, salt, cardamom, bay leaves and ½ cinnamon stick. Fry, stirring continuously, for 3–5 minutes.
2 Add the grated cauliflower and fry for a further 3–5 minutes. Serve hot with your chosen meal.

# Turnip chips with Cajun seasoning

PHASE 1 ONWARDS | SERVES 2–3

I can honestly say that you won't miss potato chips after trying these! During the maintenance phase you can have some ketchup or mayonnaise on the side, but you may not even want them, as these chips have so much flavour.

— **2 turnips, peeled**
— **30g butter**
— **2 tsp Cajun seasoning**
— **chopped fresh flat-leaf parsley, to garnish**

## HOW TO PREPARE

1 Preheat the oven to 220°C.
2 Cut each peeled turnip into a cube, then slice each turnip into square slices. Finally, cut the squares into chips.
3 Place the butter on a baking tray and put it in the oven. Once the butter has melted, add the turnip chips and Cajun seasoning. Bake in the oven for 20–30 minutes, depending on their size. Garnish with the chopped fresh parsley.

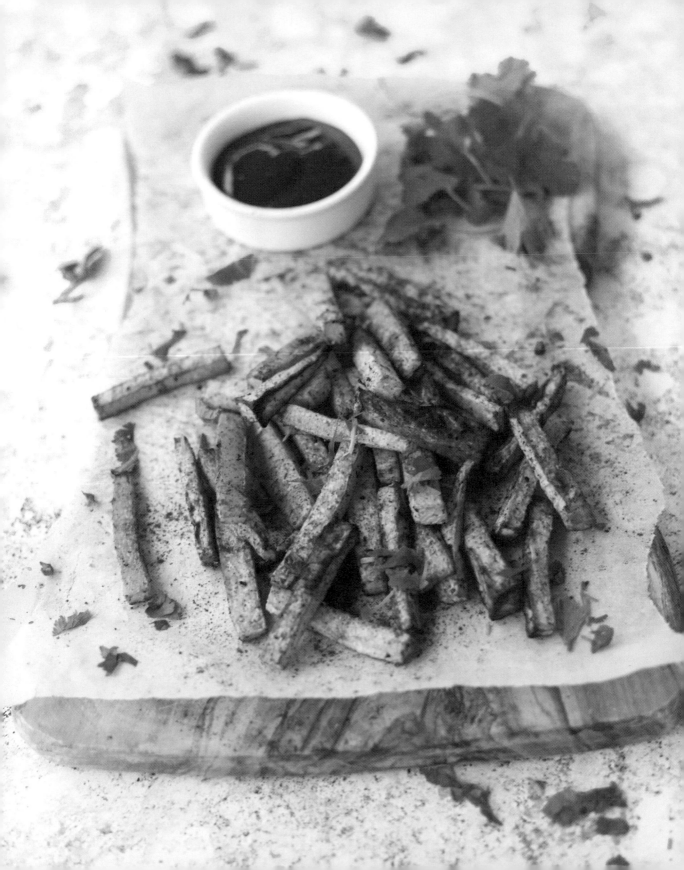

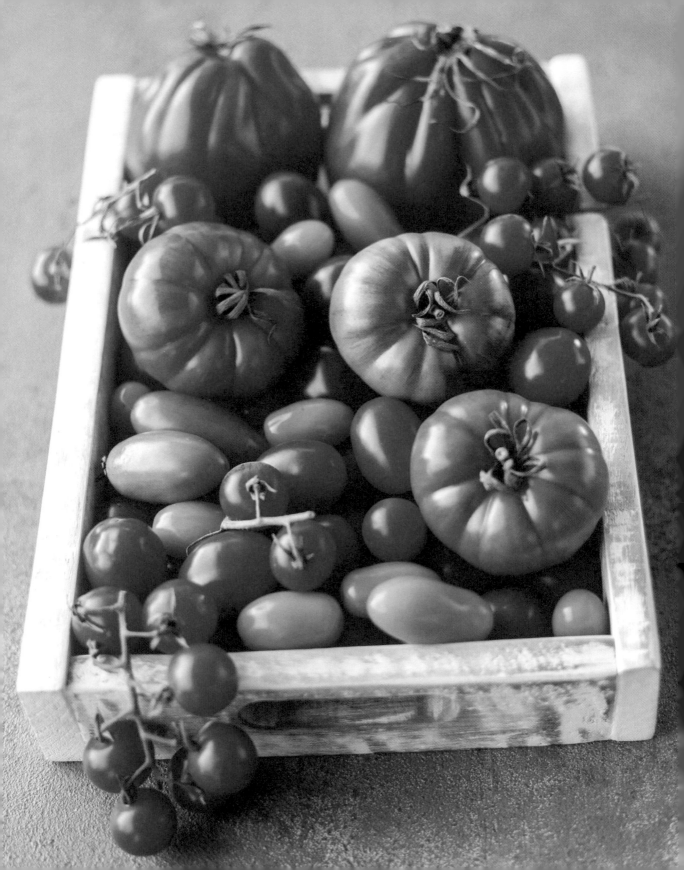

# VEGETABLE SIDE DISHES

# Aubergine pizzas

PHASE 1 ONWARDS | MAKES 9

Everyone loves a pizza! You can enjoy these pizzas as a snack or with a side salad at lunchtime instead of soup. The quality of the tinned tomatoes can make a huge difference. I have found the Mutti finely chopped tomatoes to be the best. They contain no added tomato juice or sugar.

— **1 aubergine**
— **Herbamare salt**
— **5 spring onions, green parts only, finely chopped**
— **400g tin of Mutti finely chopped tomatoes**
— **⅓ cube of Kallo tomato and herb stock (or beef stock)**
— **9 mini light mozzarella balls (available in Lidl)**
— **fresh basil leaves, to garnish**

HOW TO PREPARE

1 Cut the aubergine into 9 rounds 1cm thick (discard the very small end pieces). Place the aubergine rounds on kitchen paper. Sprinkle with Herbamare salt and leave for 10 minutes to allow the salt to draw out the excess water. After 10 minutes, turn them over and salt the other side, leaving them for another 5 minutes.

2 Now start the sauce. Place the spring onions and tinned tomatoes in a large non-stick frying pan, then crumble in the ⅓ stock cube. Cook on a high heat for 10 minutes, stirring frequently. Make sure there are no larger pieces of tomato – the sauce needs to be smooth.

3 Preheat the oven to 190°C. Line a large baking tray with non-stick baking paper.

4 While the sauce is cooking, squeeze all the excess water off the mini mozzarella balls using kitchen paper. Slice each ball into four rounds and set aside.

5 Once the aubergines are ready, gently squeeze any excess water and salt off each piece using kitchen paper. Place them on the lined baking tray and bake on the top rack of the oven for 10 minutes, turning halfway through.

6 Remove the aubergines from the oven. Place some sauce and four mozzarella slices on top of each one. Return to the oven and cook for 10 minutes, until the cheese has melted. Garnish with fresh basil leaves.

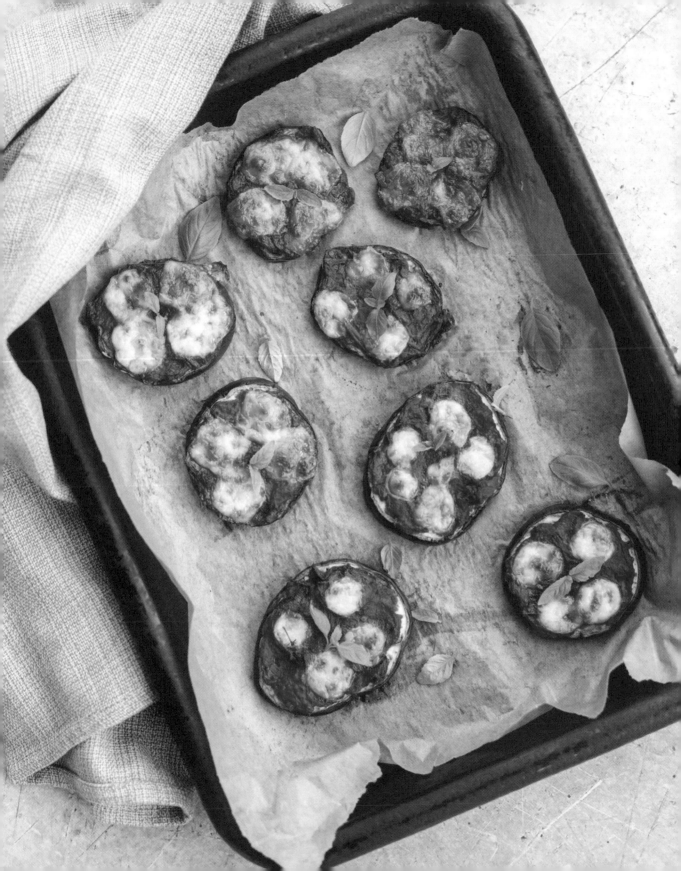

# Italian-style roasted balsamic vegetables

PHASE 1 ONWARDS | SERVES 4

You can roast many of the allowed vegetables. This is just one example of what to try and how to season them. You could try fennel instead of the courgette – just cut it into chunky slices. If you're not a fan of aubergines, swap it for a bunch of asparagus. The options are endless. Serve this as a side dish to your source of protein.

— 1 aubergine, peeled and chopped
— 1 courgette, chopped
— 1 green pepper, chopped
— 1 red pepper, chopped
— 4 garlic cloves, crushed
— 2 tbsp olive oil
— 1 tbsp Italian seasoning
— 3 ripe tomatoes, each cut into 6 pieces
— 70ml balsamic vinegar

## HOW TO PREPARE

1 Preheat the oven to 180°C.
2 Place the aubergine, courgette, peppers and garlic in a roasting tin. Add the olive oil and Italian seasoning and rub them into the vegetables using your hands. Place in the oven and roast for 20 minutes.
3 Remove the tin from the oven and add the tomatoes and balsamic vinegar. Mix well and return to the oven to roast for a further 10 minutes or until cooked to your liking.

# Tomato and vegetable sauce

PHASE 1 ONWARDS | SERVES 2

You can vary the vegetables in this sauce to suit your preferences – and the contents of your fridge. Feel free to swap the courgette for more spinach or try mushrooms instead of the green pepper. If you serve it with the Eurodiet pasta, burgers or frankfurters, they contain the protein required to make this a complete meal. You can use this sauce with meatballs or some chicken from Phase 2 onwards and swap the leek for onions when you're at the maintenance stage.

— **½ beef stock cube**

— **1 tbsp olive oil**

— **1 leek, white part only, thinly sliced**

— **2 garlic cloves, crushed**

— **1 small green pepper, diced**

— **1 celery stick, chopped**

— **½ courgette, chopped small**

— **400g tin of chopped tomatoes**

— **200g baby spinach**

— **10 fresh basil leaves, finely chopped**

— **1 tbsp tomato purée**

— **2 tsp apple cider vinegar**

— **½ tsp xylitol**

HOW TO PREPARE

1 Dissolve the beef stock cube in 60ml of boiling water.
2 Heat the oil in a deep saucepan. Add the leek and garlic and sauté for 3 minutes. Add the pepper, celery and courgette, then pour in the stock and simmer for 5 minutes.
3 Add the tinned tomatoes, spinach, fresh basil, tomato purée, apple cider vinegar and xylitol to the sauce, then simmer for 20 minutes. Serve with Eurodiet pasta to make a complete meal.

# Moroccan spiced vegetables

PHASE 1 ONWARDS | SERVES 2–4

A few years ago I got to experience authentic Moroccan cuisine during a trip to Marrakesh. I can't even describe the amazing smells and sights of the food in the markets – it was like nothing I had ever experienced before. You can buy ingredients there that many of us have never used, such as ras el hanout, which is a mixture of spices that you could use instead of the various spices listed in this recipe. Luckily for you, there's no need to travel far for this spice mix, as it is now commonly sold in large supermarkets.

- 80g green beans
- 10 cherry tomatoes, halved
- 1 aubergine, finely chopped
- 1 courgette, finely chopped
- 1 yellow pepper, finely chopped
- 1 green pepper, finely chopped
- 2 tbsp olive oil

**FOR THE SPICE MIX:**
- 2 garlic cloves, crushed
- 1 tbsp olive oil
- 2 tsp paprika
- 1 tsp xylitol
- 1 tsp sea salt
- 1 tsp ground cumin
- ½ tsp ground coriander
- ½ tsp ground turmeric
- ¼ tsp ground ginger
- ¼ tsp ground cinnamon
- ⅛ tsp cayenne pepper

HOW TO PREPARE

1 Put all the ingredients for the spice mix in a large bowl, then add the vegetables and pour in the 2 tablespoons of olive oil. Rub the spices on the vegetables using your hands. Leave to marinate for 30 minutes, or longer if possible.
2 Preheat the oven to 180°C.
3 Transfer the vegetables to a roasting tin, then roast in the oven for 30 minutes.

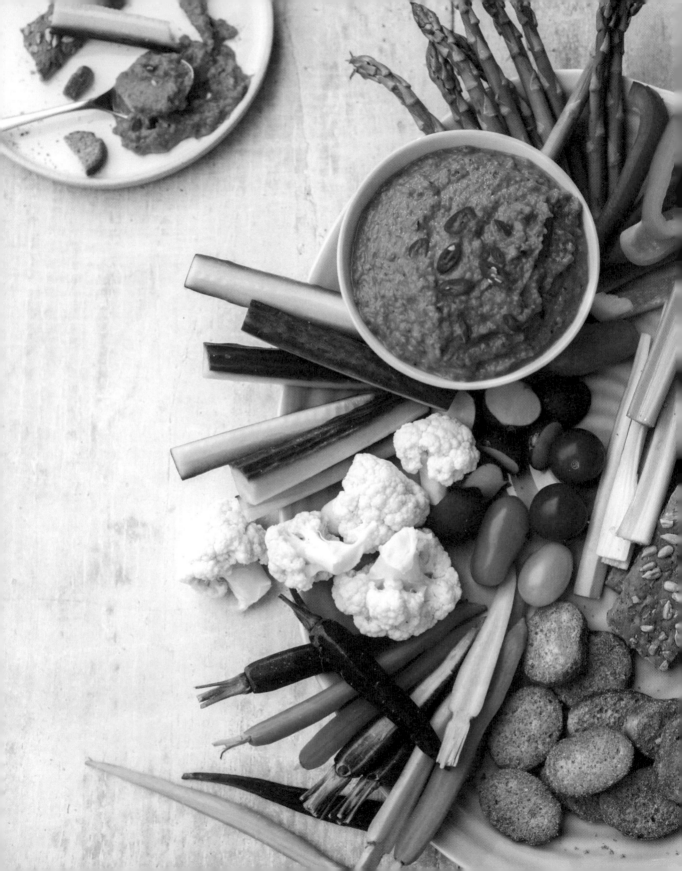

# Mediterranean vegetable dip

PHASE 1 ONWARDS | MAKES 600ML

HOW TO PREPARE

This is a clever way to eat vegetables with more vegetables! This dip has a similar consistency to hummus, but without the calories. Did you know that just 50g of hummus (typically a quarter of a standard supermarket pack) contains over 150 calories? Try this dip with cucumber and celery sticks during the early stages of your plan or use it as a spread on Eurodiet crackers. Later on, once you have reintroduced higher-carbohydrate vegetables, you can also enjoy it with carrots or sugar snap peas.

— **2 Ramiro sweet red peppers, cut into large chunks**
— **1 aubergine, peeled and cut into cubes**
— **1 courgette, halved and cut into half-circles**
— **3 garlic cloves, peeled**
— **2 tbsp olive oil**
— **1 tsp vegetable bouillon**
— **40g (approximately 2 tablespoons) Cavabel red pepper cream cheese (available in Lidl)**
— **juice of ½ a lemon**
— **1 tsp spicy Herbamare salt (optional)**

1 Preheat the oven to 180°C.
2 Prepare all the vegetables and place in a bowl. Add the oil and vegetable bouillon and rub them into all the vegetables.
3 Place the vegetables on a baking tray. Roast in the oven for 40 minutes, stirring halfway through. Remove from the tray and allow the vegetables to cool down.
4 Once the vegetables are cool, place them in a mixing bowl with the cream cheese and lemon juice. Pulse with a hand-held blender until smooth. Taste for salt and add the Herbamare if desired. Store in the fridge in an airtight container for up to three days.

# Yellow vegetable curry with curly kale

PHASE 1 ONWARDS | SERVES 1

Various curry pastes are a staple in my fridge. They can bring even the most boring vegetable stir-fry to a whole new level. Many of my clients have never tried them because they don't like curry, but trust me, they are nothing like a curry powder. You should now be able to find a variety of the flavours from all large supermarkets. A small amount of any of them goes a long way. You can serve this with konjac rice or cauliflower rice for extra bite.

— 1 tbsp coconut oil
— 1 leek, washed and thinly sliced
— 1 tbsp yellow curry paste
— 2 green peppers, thinly sliced
— 2 yellow peppers, thinly sliced
— 2 courgettes, cut into cubes
— 12 kale leaves, chopped finely
— 1 tbsp sugar-free soy sauce
— 1 tbsp oyster sauce
— 160ml full-fat coconut milk

HOW TO PREPARE

1 Heat the oil in a non-stick pan. Add the leek and curry paste and sauté for 3 minutes. Add the peppers, courgettes and kale. Keep stirring and add a splash of hot water as required to stop the vegetables from sticking.
2 Cook for 5–8 minutes, until the vegetables are cooked to your liking, then season with the soy and oyster sauces. Pour in the coconut milk, stir well and heat thoroughly before serving.

# Stir-fry with turmeric and chilli

SERVES 1

HOW TO PREPARE

Turmeric adds a beautiful colour and flavour to dishes, but be warned, it can colour anything from your hands to your tablecloths! Some supermarkets and health food shops now stock fresh turmeric root rather than just the ground version. Turmeric has become known for its health-boosting properties, especially from a substance it contains called curcumin. Enjoy this stir-fry from Phase 1 onwards and feel free to serve it with the pilau cauliflower rice (page 201) or konjac rice for additional bulk.

— 1 tsp coconut oil
— ½ bunch of spring onions, chopped
— ½ fresh red chilli, deseeded and finely chopped (optional)
— 1 tsp any curry paste
— 1 green pepper, thinly sliced
— 150g button mushrooms
— 100g bean sprouts
— 1 tsp vegetable bouillon
— freshly grated or ground turmeric, to taste

1 Heat the oil in a large frying pan or wok. Add the spring onions, chilli (if using) and curry paste. Sauté for 2 minutes, stirring constantly. Add the green pepper, mushrooms and bean sprouts and cook for 5 minutes more. Season with the vegetable bouillon and turmeric to taste.

# Stuffed courgettes

Courgettes must be one of the most versatile vegetables. You can eat them raw, they go well in stir-fries and soups and you can even replace pasta with courgetti (spiralised courgette). Grated courgettes are a great way to add volume to burgers, omelettes and even bread! In this recipe I've used them as the shells for a lovely filling. Try growing your own courgettes – they aren't difficult to grow and give a good harvest. Their beautiful flowers are also edible.

— 2 medium courgettes

— 1 tsp olive oil

— 8 mushrooms, finely chopped

— 1 leek, white part only, washed and finely chopped

— 2 garlic cloves, crushed

— 1 tsp Italian seasoning

— 1 bag of Eurodiet konjac spaghetti, rinsed well

— 120ml passata

— Herbamare salt

— freshly ground black pepper

— 10g Parmesan cheese, grated

## HOW TO PREPARE

1 Preheat the oven to 180°C.

2 Cut the ends off the courgettes and slice them in half lengthways. Using a sharp spoon, scoop out the flesh of each courgette half. Chop up the flesh and set aside to use later.

3 Bring a large saucepan of water to the boil. Place the courgette shells in the boiling water and cook for 2 minutes. Remove from the water and leave to drain in a colander.

4 While the courgette shells are cooling down, start preparing the filling. Heat the oil in a non-stick pan. Add the chopped courgette flesh, mushrooms, leek, garlic and Italian seasoning. Cook until all the vegetables have softened. Add the konjac spaghetti and passata and simmer for 2–3 minutes. Season to taste with Herbamare salt and freshly ground black pepper.

5 Place the courgette shells in an ovenproof dish. Divide the filling between the shells. Sprinkle with the Parmesan cheese and cook in the oven for 15 minutes.

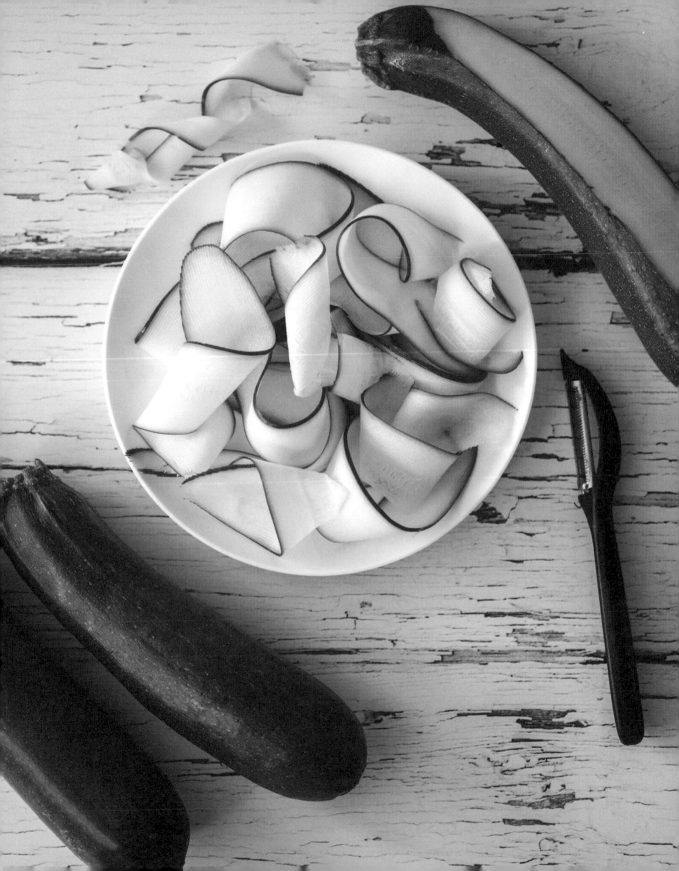

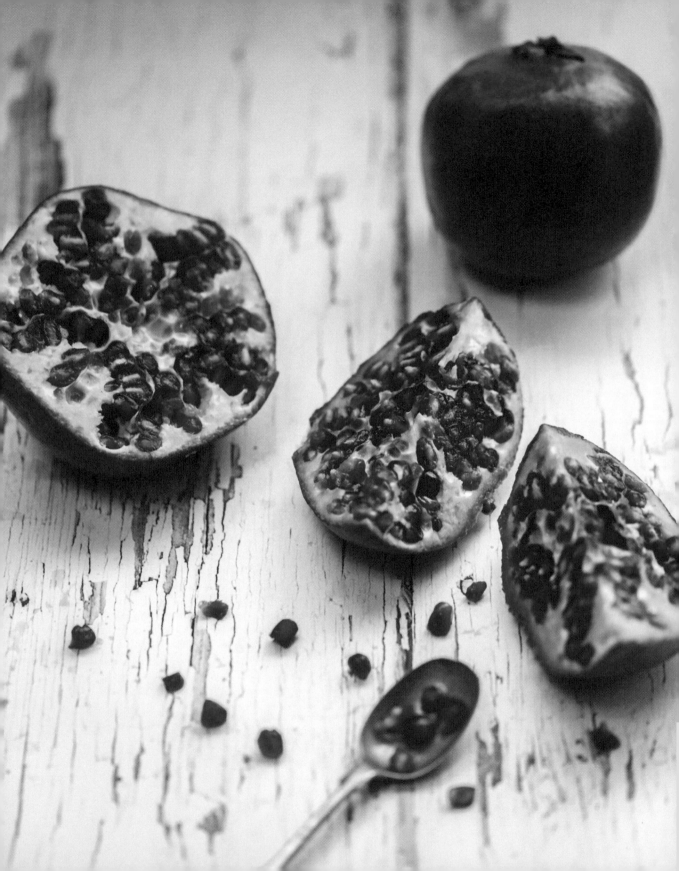

# DESSERT

# Chilled chocolate and avocado mousse

I'm a self-confessed chocoholic! There's just something so nice and satisfying about the sweetness combined with the fat that you get in an average chocolate bar. Dark chocolate is nowhere near as nice as my favourite Finnish Fazer chocolate, but it's the only one I can safely keep in my house. To me, there's no such thing as just having one square of chocolate – I will eat the whole bar, except when it comes to the darker, more bitter varieties. This dessert hits the spot due to the high fat content of the avocado and the sweetness of the banana and you can still really taste the chocolate.

— **1 small ripe banana**
— **2 frozen avocado halves**
— **60g dark chocolate (at least 85% cocoa content), plus extra for grating**
— **90ml unsweetened almond milk**
— **1 tsp vanilla extract**

## HOW TO PREPARE

1 Cut the banana into 8 small slices and place in a freezer-safe container. Freeze overnight.
2 Approximately 2 hours before serving, take the banana and the avocado halves out of the freezer. Place in a NutriBullet container and set aside to defrost to the point where they're still chilled but not too hard for the NutriBullet.
3 Place the chocolate and almond milk in a microwave-proof bowl. Microwave for 30 seconds at 900W and stir until the chocolate melts evenly into the milk. Pour this immediately into the NutriBullet container. Add the vanilla extract and blend until smooth.
4 Divide the mousse between two serving dishes and top with extra grated chocolate. Enjoy chilled.

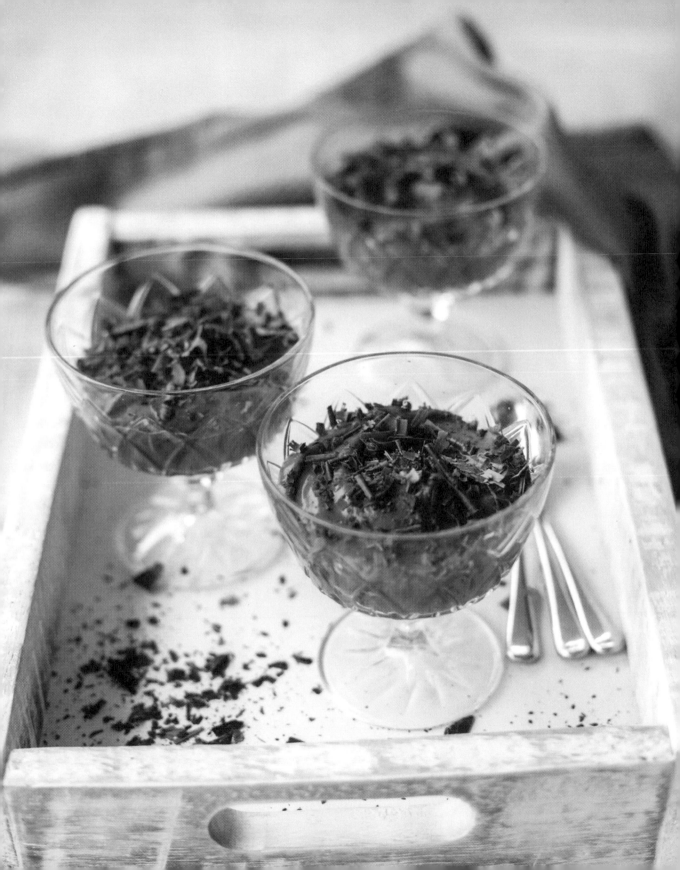

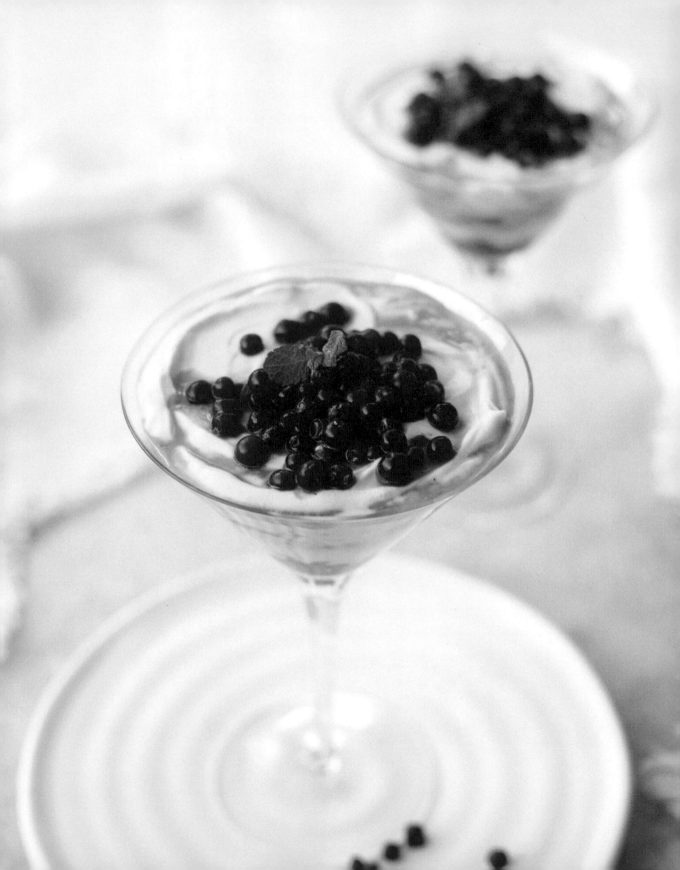

# Creamy cowberry and quark dessert

Cowberry (also known as lingonberry) is a native of my home country, Finland. It tastes a bit bitter, but xylitol will give it some sweetness. In Ireland you can find frozen cowberries in Polish food shops or you can substitute them with raspberries or blueberries. If you are using frozen berries, take them out to thaw in the fridge a few hours before making this dessert. I use quark, the fat-free yet low-sugar alternative to soft cheese, to keep the calories down and increase the protein.

— **200ml whipping cream**
— **250g quark cheese**
— **1 tsp vanilla extract**
— **200g cowberries, blueberries or raspberries**
— **xylitol, to taste**
— **small sprigs of fresh mint, to decorate**

## HOW TO PREPARE

1 Whip the cream using an electric whisk until peaks form. Add the quark and vanilla extract. Check the flavour and add some xylitol to sweeten it if desired.
2 Layer four serving glasses with the mixture and the berries and decorate with a small sprig of fresh mint on top. Serve chilled.

# Lemon and raspberry cheesecakes

PHASE 1 ONWARDS | MAKES 4 MINI
CHEESECAKES (2 PER PORTION)

These cheesecakes are a big hit amongst
my patients when they want to either
bring something to a party or are hosting
one themselves. One serving has only a
fraction of the calories and sugar that
a slice of traditional cheesecake would
contain. Try them for yourself instead
of just taking my word for it – they
are delicious.

— ½ sachet of gelatine (5.5g)
— 3 Eurodiet raspberry biscuits
— 1 tsp coconut oil
— 100g good-quality thick Greek yoghurt
— 50g ricotta cheese
— 3 tbsp lemon juice
— 1 tsp xylitol or stevia
— 4 tsp unwaxed lemon zest

## HOW TO PREPARE

1 Dissolve the ½ sachet of gelatine in
250ml of boiling water. Set aside to let
the water cool down.

2 Place the biscuits in a freezer bag and
close it. Crush the biscuits into fine
crumbs with a rolling pin.

3 Heat the coconut oil in the microwave
for approximately 30 seconds, until
melted. Add the crushed biscuits to
the melted oil and mix well. Divide this
mixture between four silicone cupcake
holders. Press the mixture down
towards the bottom of the cupcake
holders and place them in the fridge.

4 Put the yoghurt, ricotta cheese, lemon
juice and xylitol into a medium-sized
bowl. Add 3 teaspoons of the lemon
zest, keeping 1 teaspoon for decoration.
Mix well.

5 Add the cold gelatine mixture to the
ricotta and yoghurt mixture and mix well.
Divide this mix between the cupcake
holders with the cooled biscuit base. Chill
in the fridge for approximately 6 hours,
until set, or overnight. Decorate with the
remaining teaspoon of lemon zest.

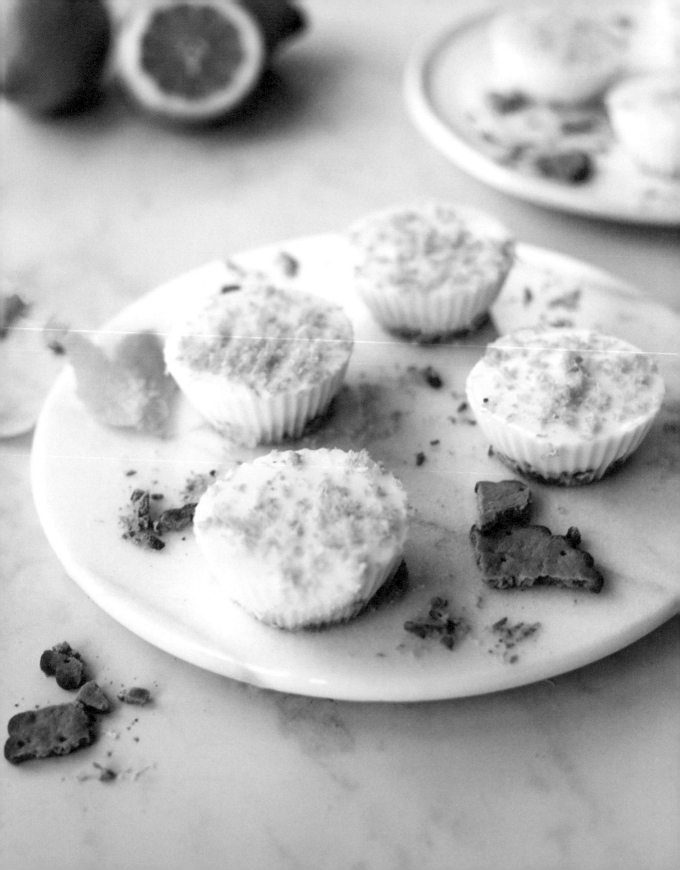

# Strawberry and vanilla trifle

MAINTENANCE | MAKES 2 SMALL TRIFLES
(SERVES 2)

It's so important to be able to have a
nice treat during your diet. People are
more likely to succeed when the changes
they are expected to make are not huge
right from the start. I've met many
people who are determined to do the diet
without anything that resembles a treat,
but typically they only have this level of
enthusiasm for a week or two. Without a
nice dessert like this, you might be more
likely to cheat, then feel like a failure and
give up. Losing weight and taking control of
your diabetes is a journey, so treat yourself
a little if it helps you to get to the end goal!

— **1 Eurodiet muffin**
— **1 sachet of Hartley's strawberry sugar-free jelly
   crystals (11g)**
— **1 Laktolight sachet**
— **1 packet of Eurodiet vanilla dessert**

HOW TO PREPARE

1 Slice the Eurodiet muffin into six pieces
  and divide between two glass trifle
  dishes.
2 Dissolve the sachet of jelly crystals in
  300ml of boiling water. Once dissolved,
  top up with a further 200ml of cold
  water. Pour the jelly into the glass
  dishes over the muffins. Place the
  dishes in the fridge to allow the jelly
  to set.
3 Once the jelly has set, fill your shaker
  with 150ml of cold water. Empty the
  Laktolight sachet into it and shake
  well. Empty the vanilla dessert sachet
  into the Laktolight milk and shake well
  again. Leave the mixture to stand for
  4 minutes.
4 Divide the dessert between the two
  glasses and serve.

# Appendix: Alternative Products to Eurodiet

In my clinics we use Eurodiet products for a number of reasons. The range has a lot of variety, which means you're not as likely to get fed up and go off the diet. All Eurodiet products (at the time of going to print) are also supplemented with protein, vitamins, minerals and fibre, with the exception of konjac rice and konjac noodles which contain no nutritional value except fibre. I have included the Eurodiet range in my meal plans and recipes simply because they are the range that I have the most experience with, so I know that the products work.

There are a number of other products on the market, which I have listed below. There may well be other products available, but these are the ones I have come across. However, a word of caution! If you are looking for alternative products to the Eurodiet range to use on the VLCKD, make sure to compare the protein, carbohydrate, vitamin, mineral and fibre content. Having looked at the nutritional information on some of the products available, the carbohydrate and sugar content is significantly higher than that of the Eurodiet product range.

- MyProtein Very Low Calorie Diet Meal Replacement (VLCD). Available online only. MyProtein offers bars, drinks, breakfasts, desserts, shakes, meals.
- The Cambridge weight-loss plan offers a variety of bars, drinks, smoothies, shakes, soups, breakfasts and complete savoury meals. To use these products you must be using a Cambridge Weight Plan and see a consultant first.
- The Exante diet offers a range of shakes, breakfast options, bars, complete meals, soups and desserts for weight loss.

# INDEX

## A

alcohol 48–9, 69
alfalfa, Cloud bread with smoked salmon and avocado 105
allicin 122
almond milk, Chilled chocolate and avocado mousse 220
almonds (ground), Fish cakes 184
Alzheimer's disease 42–3
apple cider vinegar
    Raw power salad with strawberry vinaigrette 119
    Tomato and vegetable sauce 209
apples, Beetroot salad 145
artichokes 60
asparagus 97
    Asparagus and blue cheese soup 134
    Eurodiet omelette 102
aubergines 60, 97
    Aubergine pizzas 206
    Chicken and aubergine bake 176
    Italian-style roasted balsamic vegetables 208
    Mediterranean vegetable dip 213
    Moroccan spiced vegetables 210–11
    Moussaka 181
avocados
    Chilled chocolate and avocado mousse 220
    Cloud bread with smoked salmon and avocado 105

## B

bacon
    Beef and red wine casserole 187
    Spaghetti carbonara 163
balsamic vinegar
    Beetroot salad 145
    Italian-style roasted balsamic vegetables 208
bananas, Chilled chocolate and avocado mousse 220
basil
    Aubergine pizzas 206
    Creamy vegetable soup 138
    Eurodiet pasta salad with pesto 122
    Pea and herb soup 140
    Tomato and vegetable sauce 209

bean sprouts 97
    Pork in black bean sauce 170
    Stir-fry with turmeric and chilli 215
beans 60, 97
    Chilli sin carne 177
    Moroccan spiced vegetables 210–11
    Pork in black bean sauce 170
    Tomato and bean soup 139
beef 80
    Beef and red wine casserole 187
    Moussaka 181
    Pasta Bolognese 164
Beetroot salad 145
black pudding, Hunter's casserole 188
blue cheese
    Asparagus and blue cheese soup 134
    Buffalo chicken wrap pizza 131
BMI (body mass index) 35, 44, 62, 88
    vs waist measurement 38–40
BMR (basal metabolic rate) 89, 91
bread
    Cloud bread with smoked salmon and avocado 105
    Eurodiet bread 120
British Medical Journal 41
broccoli 60, 97
    Vegetable gratin 197
brown rice 84
    Yellow peppers stuffed with feta and pine nuts 191
Buffalo chicken wrap pizza 131
butternut squash, Vegetarian burgers with tzatziki and quinoa 182–3

## C

cabbage 60, 97
    Celeriac and cabbage slaw 146
    Yuk sung with spicy cabbage 159–61
calories
    alcoholic drinks and 49
    BMR and 89
    energy balance and 88
    Eurodiet products and 73
    FSAI daily recommendation 88
    GDAs and 88
Cambridge Weight Plan 227
Cape Malay-style fish curry 186
carbohydrates
    breakfast and 84
    dinner and 84
    Eurodiet products and 73
    GI (glycaemic index) and 90

    glucose control and 84–5
    low-GI 90
    lunch and 84
    portion sizes 84
    slow-releasing (low GI) 26
    substitutes 196–202
    VLCKD maintenance phase and 87–8
    VLCKD Plan and 72, 84
    weight and 91–2
carrots 60
    Chilli sin carne 177
    Hunter's casserole 188
    Tomato and bean soup 139
cauliflower 60, 96, 97
    Cauliflower and celery soup with spices 135
    Cauliflower rice 196
    Chorizo and cauliflower soup 137
    Pilau cauliflower rice 201
    Raw power salad with strawberry vinaigrette 119
    Vegetable gratin 197
celeriac 97
    Celeriac and cabbage slaw 146
    Sweet potato and celeriac soup 144
    Vegetable gratin 197
celery 97
    Beef and red wine casserole 187
    Cauliflower and celery soup with spices 135
    Hunter's casserole 188
    Spicy chicken and vegetable casserole 158
    Tomato and bean soup 139
    Tomato and vegetable sauce 209
    Yuk sung with spicy cabbage 159–61
Cheddar cheese
    Buffalo chicken wrap pizza 131
    Chicken fajitas 192
    Eurodiet pizza 154
    Moussaka 181
cheeses 98, 99
    see also blue cheese; Cheddar cheese; cream cheese; feta cheese; mozzarella cheese; Parmesan cheese; quark cheese; ricotta cheese
chia seeds, Eurodiet strawberry chia pudding 109
chicken
    Buffalo chicken wrap pizza 131
    Chicken and aubergine bake 176
    Chicken Caesar lettuce wrap 147

Chicken fajitas 192
Chicken and turnip curry 167
Spicy chicken and vegetable
  casserole 158
Warm chicken and coconut
  salad 130
chickpeas
  Tomato and bean soup 139
  Vegetarian burgers with tzatziki
    and quinoa 182–3
Chilled chocolate and avocado
  mousse 220
Chilli sin carne 177
chillis
  Cauliflower and celery soup with
    spices 135
  Celeriac and cabbage slaw 146
  Finn Crisp rolls with cream
    cheese 125
  Fish cakes 184
  Jambalaya 172
  Stir-fry with turmeric and chilli
    215
  Yuk sung with spicy cabbage
    159–61
chives, Frittata breakfast cups 113
chocolate, Chilled chocolate and
  avocado mousse 220
chorizo
  Chorizo and cauliflower soup 137
  Jambalaya 172
Cloud bread with smoked salmon and
  avocado 105
coconut (desiccated), Warm chicken
  and coconut salad 130
coconut milk
  Cauliflower and celery soup with
    spices 135
  Chicken and turnip curry 167
  Yellow vegetable curry with curly
    kale 214
constipation 70–1
coriander (fresh)
  Cape Malay-style fish curry 186
  Cauliflower and celery soup with
    spices 135
  Chicken fajitas 192
  Chicken and turnip curry 167
  Chilli sin carne 177
  Fish cakes 184
  Jambalaya 172
  Prawns with konjac spaghetti 171
courgettes 60, 96, 97
  Chicken and aubergine bake 176
  Creamy vegetable soup 138
  Eurodiet frittata 153

Eurodiet pasta salad with
  pesto 122
Italian-style roasted balsamic
  vegetables 208
Lamb and feta burgers 168
Mediterranean vegetable dip 213
Moroccan spiced vegetables
  210–11
Moussaka 181
Pasta Bolognese 164
Pea and herb soup 140
Spicy chicken and vegetable
  casserole 158
Stuffed courgettes 216
Tomato and vegetable sauce 209
Yellow vegetable curry with curly
  kale 214
cowberries, Creamy cowberry and
quark dessert 223
cream cheese
  Chorizo and cauliflower soup 137
  Cloud bread with smoked
    salmon and avocado 105
  Eurodiet pasta salad with
    pesto 122
  Finn Crisp rolls with cream
    cheese 125
  Mediterranean vegetable dip 213
  Mushroom risotto with konjac
    rice 198
  Spicy chicken and vegetable
    casserole 158
  Vegetable gratin 197
Creamy cowberry and quark dessert
  223
Creamy mushroom soup 142
Creamy vegetable soup 138
crème fraîche, Fish cakes 184
crispbreads
  Finn Crisp rolls with cream
    cheese 125
  Vegetarian burgers with tzatziki
    and quinoa 182–3
cucumbers 60, 97
  Finn Crisp rolls with cream
    cheese 125
  Vegetarian burgers with tzatziki
    and quinoa 182–3
curry paste
  Chicken and turnip curry 167
  Eurodiet egg fried rice 150
  Prawns with konjac spaghetti 171
  Stir-fry with turmeric and chilli
    215
  Sweet potato and celeriac soup
    144

Yellow vegetable curry with curly
  kale 214
Yuk sung with spicy cabbage
  159–61

**D**

diabetes case studies
  Burke, Terry 27–9
  Cheevers, Peggy 17–18, 62
  Coyne, Brendan 23–6, 34, 38, 67
  Dalton, John 16–17, 22, 34
  Delaney, Joan 11–13, 32
  Kelly, James 19–20, 67
  Miss J 14–15, 39, 40, 62
  Mulcahy, Pat 30–1, 67
  Treacy, Tom 21–2
diabetes in Ireland 4–6
diabetes mellitus (T1DM) 5, 33, 36,
  37, 38
diabetes mellitus (T2DM) 33–4
  abdominal obesity and 4
  activity levels and 42
  age and 41
  alcohol and 48–9
  Alzheimer's disease and 42–3
  bad diet and 41
  blood glucose checks 50, 51
  cancer and 43, 54
  causes of 4, 7, 41–2
  chain of causation 7
  chronic inflammation and 40–2
  complications associated with
    5–6, 10, 21, 22
  definition 7, 32
  diagnosis 36
  diet and 10
  driving and 50–1
  GGT levels 48
  glucose levels, infections and
    37–8
  HbA1c level 44–6, 54, 84–5
  hypoglycaemic episodes 23, 25,
    34, 38, 50–1
  IDF guidelines 53
  insulin injections and 24, 30
  insulin resistance and 4, 25, 34,
    37, 38, 43
  life expectancy and 10
  Long-Term Illness Scheme
    and 6
  medical solution 34
  medication, side effects of 41
  metabolic programming and 42
  obesity and 34
  obstructive sleep apnoea and
    43–4

smoking and 47
symptom-led medicine and 40
symptoms 34
thirst and 30
TOFI 11, 12, 35, 39
treatment of 10
visceral fat and 34, 35, 36, 39, 40
weight and 4, 10, 34
diabetes mellitus (Type 3) 42
diabetes/pre-diabetes 32, 45, 46
diabetic ketoacidosis (DKA) 36, 37
diabetic medication
 Amaryl 56–7
 aspirin 21
 Atorvastatin 17
 beta cell degeneration and 55, 56
 Bydureon 58–9
 Byetta 58–9
 combinations of 55
 Diaclide MR 56
 Diamicron 30, 37–8, 50, 55, 56–7
 DPP4-inhibitors 54, 55, 58–9
 Eucreas 21, 22
 Forxiga 56
 glibenclamides/glyburides 54
 Glucophage 11, 12, 14, 22, 30,
  56–7
 Humalog 58–9
 hypoglycaemia, risk of 54, 56
 IDF guidelines 53
 incretin mimetics 58–9
 insulin 58–9
 Invokana 56–7
 Janumet 55
 Januvia 58–9
 Jardiance 56–7
 Lantus 58–9
 Levemir 58–9
 Metformin 11, 21, 45, 50, 55, 56–7
 Metformin Mylan 56–7
 Nexium 21
 Novorapid 58–9
 Ramipril 17
 SGLT2 inhibitors 55, 56–7
 side effects 14, 53–60, 66
 statins 17, 21
 sulphonylurea 37–8, 50, 54, 55,
  56–7
 Synjardy 17, 18, 55
 Trajenta 18, 58–9
 Tresiba 58–9
 Trulicity 58–9
 Victoza 58–9
 Warfarin (Coumadin) 60
 weight gain and 55, 65

**D**

Dijon mustard, Creamy mushroom
 soup 142
DiRECT study 4
driving, diabetes and 50–1

**E**

eggs 80
 Cloud bread with smoked
  salmon and avocado 105
 Frittata breakfast cups 113
 Spaghetti carbonara 163
 Vegetarian burgers with tzatziki
  and quinoa 182–3
 Warm chicken and coconut
  salad 130
Eurodiet biscuits, Lemon and
 raspberry cheesecakes 224
Eurodiet bread 120
Eurodiet croutons
 Chicken Caesar lettuce wrap 147
 Pea and herb soup 140
Eurodiet egg fried rice 150
Eurodiet frittata 153
Eurodiet konjac rice
 Eurodiet egg fried rice 150
 Eurodiet rice pudding 110
 Jambalaya 172
 Mushroom risotto with konjac
  rice 198
 Pork in black bean sauce 170
 Stuffed tomatoes 156
Eurodiet konjac spaghetti
 Pasta Bolognese 164
 Prawns with konjac spaghetti 171
 Spaghetti carbonara 163
 Stuffed courgettes 216
Eurodiet muffin, Strawberry and
 vanilla trifle 226
Eurodiet omelette sachet
 Eurodiet frittata 153
 Eurodiet omelette 102
Eurodiet pasta salad with pesto 122
Eurodiet pizza 154
Eurodiet porridge with stewed
 rhubarb 106–8
Eurodiet products 28, 63–4, 72, 73
 alternative products 227
Eurodiet rice pudding 110
Eurodiet strawberry chia pudding 109
Eurodiet strawberry spread, Raw
 power salad with strawberry
 vinaigrette 119

Eurodiet vanilla dessert, Strawberry
 and vanilla trifle 226
Eurodiet vegetarian Bolognese sachet,
 Stuffed tomatoes 156
European Association for the Study of
 Diabetes (EASD) 46
Extante diet 227

**F**

FDA (Food and Drug Administration)
 54, 56, 58
feta cheese
 Frittata breakfast cups 113
 Lamb and feta burgers 168
 Spaghetti carbonara 163
 Yellow peppers stuffed with feta
  and pine nuts 191
fibre 60, 64, 70, 72, 73, 90
Fiery pizza with spicy pepperoni and
 jalapeño peppers 178–9
Finland 5, 198, 223
fish 80
 Cape Malay-style fish curry 186
 Cloud bread with smoked
  salmon and avocado 105
 Fish cakes 184
fish sauce
 Prawns with konjac spaghetti 171
 Yuk sung with spicy cabbage
  159–61
flaxseeds, Eurodiet bread 120
food pyramids 7, 8, 9, 10, 61
Food Safety Authority of Ireland
 (FSAI) 88
Frittata breakfast cups 113
fructose 130
fruit 84
fruit juices 10

**G**

garlic
 Asparagus and blue cheese soup
  134
 Beef and red wine casserole 187
 Cape Malay-style fish curry 186
 Cauliflower and celery soup with
  spices 135
 Celeriac and cabbage slaw 146
 Chicken and aubergine bake 176
 Chicken fajitas 192
 Chicken and turnip curry 167
 Creamy vegetable soup 138
 Eurodiet pasta salad with pesto
  122

Green lentil and pomegranate
molasses salad 126–8
Hunter's casserole 188
Italian-style roasted balsamic
vegetables 208
Jambalaya 172
Mediterranean vegetable dip 213
Moroccan spiced vegetables
210–11
Moussaka 181
Pilau cauliflower rice 201
Stuffed courgettes 216
Tomato and vegetable sauce 209
Vegetarian burgers with tzatziki
and quinoa 182–3
Vegetarian lasagne 190
Yuk sung with spicy cabbage
159–61
gelatine, Lemon and raspberry
cheesecakes 224
gherkins 97
Beef and red wine casserole 187
Turkey and horseradish burgers
175
ginger
Eurodiet egg fried rice 150
Prawns with konjac spaghetti 171
Sweet potato and celeriac soup
144
Yuk sung with spicy cabbage
159–61
glycaemic index (GI) 90
Green lentil and pomegranate
molasses salad 126–8
Guinness, Hunter's casserole 188

**H**

ham, Frittata breakfast cups 113
Herbamare salt
Aubergine pizzas 206
Beef and red wine casserole 187
Celeriac and cabbage slaw 146
Chicken and aubergine bake 176
Chicken fajitas 192
Eurodiet pasta salad with pesto
122
Mediterranean vegetable dip 213
Pea and herb soup 140
Raw power salad with strawberry
vinaigrette 119
Spicy chicken and vegetable
casserole 158
Stuffed courgettes 216
Turkey and horseradish burgers
175

Vegetarian burgers with tzatziki
and quinoa 182–3
Warm chicken and coconut
salad 130
herbs (dried)
Cauliflower rice 196
Eurodiet omelette 102
Fish cakes 184
Spaghetti carbonara 163
Vegetarian lasagne 190
herbs (fresh)
Beef and red wine casserole 187
Eurodiet frittata 153
Hunter's casserole 188
Lamb and feta burgers 168
see also basil; chives; coriander
(fresh); mint; parsley (flat-
leaf)
hormones 33, 38, 40, 42, 65–6
cortisol 69–70, 91
horseradish, Turkey and horseradish
burgers 175
hot pepper sauce
Buffalo chicken wrap pizza 131
Chicken and aubergine bake 176
Fiery pizza with spicy pepperoni
and jalapeño peppers 178–9
Prawns with konjac spaghetti 171
Spicy chicken and vegetable
casserole 158
Stuffed tomatoes 156
Hunter's casserole 188

**I**

IDF Diabetes Atlas 5
International Diabetes Federation
(IDF) 4, 53, 54–5
Italian-style roasted balsamic
vegetables 208

**J**

jalapeños, Fiery pizza with spicy
pepperoni and jalapeño peppers
178–9
Jambalaya 172
jelly, Strawberry and vanilla trifle 226
Jenkins, David 90

**K**

kaffir lime leaves, Chicken and turnip
curry 167
kale 97
Yellow vegetable curry with curly
kale 214

kefir, Tropical breakfast smoothie 114
ketoacidosis 36, 37
ketogenic diet 37, 64–5
see also Very Low Calorie
Ketogenic Diet; VLCKD diet
plan
ketosis 2, 36–7, 72, 85
VLCKD and 65, 74, 78

**L**

Laktolight sachets 77
contraindications 77
Eurodiet bread 120
Eurodiet egg fried rice 150
Eurodiet frittata 153
Eurodiet omelette 102
Eurodiet pizza 154
Eurodiet porridge with stewed
rhubarb 106–8
Eurodiet rice pudding 110
Strawberry and vanilla trifle 226
lamb 80
Lamb and feta burgers 168
Moussaka 181
leeks 97
Asparagus and blue cheese soup
134
Cauliflower rice 196
Chicken and turnip curry 167
Creamy vegetable soup 138
Eurodiet frittata 153
Pasta Bolognese 164
Pea and herb soup 140
Pork in black bean sauce 170
Spicy chicken and vegetable
casserole 158
Stuffed courgettes 216
Tomato and vegetable sauce 209
Yellow vegetable curry with curly
kale 214
lemongrass, Sweet potato and celeriac
soup 144
lemons
Celeriac and cabbage slaw 146
Green lentil and pomegranate
molasses salad 126–8
Lemon and raspberry
cheesecakes 224
Mediterranean vegetable dip 213
lentils, Green lentil and pomegranate
molasses salad 126–8
lettuce 97
Chicken Caesar lettuce wrap 147
Chicken fajitas 192
Raw power salad with strawberry
vinaigrette 119

Turkey and horseradish burgers 175

Warm chicken and coconut salad 130

Yuk sung with spicy cabbage 159–61

limes

Celeriac and cabbage slaw 146

Chicken and turnip curry 167

Jambalaya 172

Prawns with konjac spaghetti 171

Lourens, Wilma 26

**M**

mangos, Tropical breakfast smoothie 114

matcha green tea powder, Tropical breakfast smoothie 114

mayonnaise, Celeriac and cabbage slaw 146

Mediterranean vegetable dip 213

milk 72

White sauce 190

minerals 63

Eurodiet products and 64

mint

Celeriac and cabbage slaw 146

Green lentil and pomegranate molasses salad 126–8

Pea and herb soup 140

Vegetarian burgers with tzatziki and quinoa 182–3

Moroccan spiced vegetables 210–11

Moussaka 181

mozzarella cheese

Aubergine pizzas 206

Buffalo chicken wrap pizza 131

Fiery pizza with spicy pepperoni and jalapeño peppers 178–9

Moussaka 181

Vegetarian lasagne 190

mushrooms 60, 97

Beef and red wine casserole 187

Creamy mushroom soup 142

Mushroom risotto with konjac rice 198

Pasta Bolognese 164

Pork in black bean sauce 170

Stir-fry with turmeric and chilli 215

Stuffed courgettes 216

Yuk sung with spicy cabbage 159–61

Mutti pizza sauce

Aubergine pizzas 206

Buffalo chicken wrap pizza 131

Eurodiet pizza 154

Fiery pizza with spicy pepperoni and jalapeño peppers 178–9

MyProtein Very Low Calorie Diet Meal Replacement (VLCD) 227

**O**

omega-3 fatty acids 64

omelette, Eurodiet omelette 102

onions 60

Beef and red wine casserole 187

Cape Malay-style fish curry 186

Chicken fajitas 192

Chilli sin carne 177

Green lentil and pomegranate molasses salad 126–8

Moussaka 181

Sweet potato and celeriac soup 144

Tomato and bean soup 139

Vegetarian lasagne 190

Yellow peppers stuffed with feta and pine nuts 191

see also spring onions

onions (pickled), Hunter's casserole 188

orange juice, Beetroot salad 145

oyster sauce, Yellow vegetable curry with curly kale 214

**P**

pak choi 97

Chicken and turnip curry 167

Eurodiet egg fried rice 150

Prawns with konjac spaghetti 171

Parmesan cheese

Chicken and aubergine bake 176

Eurodiet frittata 153

Green lentil and pomegranate molasses salad 126–8

Pasta Bolognese 164

Spaghetti carbonara 163

Stuffed courgettes 216

Vegetable gratin 197

parsley (flat-leaf)

Chorizo and cauliflower soup 137

Fish cakes 184

Green lentil and pomegranate molasses salad 126–8

parsnips, Tomato and bean soup 139

pasta

Eurodiet pasta salad with pesto 122

Pasta Bolognese 164

portion size 84

Vegetarian lasagne 190

peas

Cape Malay-style fish curry 186

Pea and herb soup 140

peppadews, Yellow peppers stuffed with feta and pine nuts 191

pepperoni, Fiery pizza with spicy pepperoni and jalapeño peppers 178–9

peppers 97

Chicken fajitas 192

Green lentil and pomegranate molasses salad 126–8

peppers (green) 60

Chilli sin carne 177

Eurodiet pizza 154

Italian-style roasted balsamic vegetables 208

Jambalaya 172

Moroccan spiced vegetables 210–11

Spicy chicken and vegetable casserole 158

Stir-fry with turmeric and chilli 215

Tomato and vegetable sauce 209

Yellow vegetable curry with curly kale 214

Yuk sung with spicy cabbage 159–61

peppers (orange)

Creamy vegetable soup 138

Eurodiet egg fried rice 150

Pork in black bean sauce 170

Prawns with konjac spaghetti 171

Warm chicken and coconut salad 130

peppers (red)

Chicken and turnip curry 167

Chilli sin carne 177

Italian-style roasted balsamic vegetables 208

Mediterranean vegetable dip 213

Warm chicken and coconut salad 130

Yuk sung with spicy cabbage 159–61

peppers (yellow)

Jambalaya 172

Moroccan spiced vegetables 210–11

Pork in black bean sauce 170

Yellow peppers stuffed with feta and pine nuts 191

Yellow vegetable curry with curly kale 214

pesto, Eurodiet pasta salad with
pesto 122
Pilau cauliflower rice 201
pine nuts
Eurodiet pasta salad with pesto
122
Yellow peppers stuffed with feta
and pine nuts 191
pineapple, Warm chicken and
coconut salad 130
pizza
Aubergine pizzas 206
Buffalo chicken wrap pizza 131
Eurodiet pizza 154
Fiery pizza with spicy pepperoni
and jalapeño peppers 178–9
pomegranates, Green lentil and
pomegranate molasses salad 126–8
pork 80
Pork in black bean sauce 170
Yuk sung with spicy cabbage
159–61
potatoes
Cape Malay-style fish curry 186
Fish cakes 184
prawns
Jambalaya 172
Prawns with konjac spaghetti 171
protein 48, 62, 64, 65, 80
Eurodiet products and 73
psyllium husks 70
Eurodiet bread 120

**Q**

quark cheese, Creamy cowberry and
quark dessert 223
quinoa 84
Vegetarian burgers with tzatziki
and quinoa 182–3
Quorn products 80

**R**

radishes 97
Raw power salad with
strawberry vinaigrette 119
Raw power salad with strawberry
vinaigrette 119
rhubarb 70
Eurodiet porridge with stewed
rhubarb 106–8
ricotta cheese
Creamy mushroom soup 142
Creamy vegetable soup 138
Lemon and raspberry
cheesecakes 224

Road Safety Authority (RSA) 51
rocket 97
Eurodiet frittata 153
Eurodiet pizza 154
Fiery pizza with spicy pepperoni
and jalapeño peppers 178–9
Stuffed tomatoes 156
Ryan, Mary 43

**S**

salad leaves 60
Eurodiet pasta salad with pesto
122
Eurodiet pizza 154
Raw power salad with
strawberry vinaigrette 119
Spaghetti carbonara 163
salsa (fresh)
Chicken fajitas 192
Chilli sin carne 177
sleep 91
obstructive sleep apnoea (OSA)
43–4
weight loss and 69
smoked salmon, Cloud bread with
smoked salmon and avocado 105
smoking 47
soy sauce (sugar-free)
Cape Malay-style fish curry 186
Chicken fajitas 192
Chicken and turnip curry 167
Eurodiet egg fried rice 150
Fish cakes 184
Prawns with konjac spaghetti
171
Yellow vegetable curry with
curly kale 214
Yuk sung with spicy cabbage
159–61
Spaghetti carbonara 163
spices
Cape Malay-style fish curry 186
Cauliflower and celery soup
with spices 135
Chilli sin carne 177
Jambalaya 172
Moroccan spiced vegetables
210–11
Pilau cauliflower rice 201
Stir-fry with turmeric and chilli
215
Spicy chicken and vegetable casserole
158
spinach 60, 97
Tomato and vegetable sauce 209
Vegetarian lasagne 190

Warm chicken and coconut
salad 130
spring onions 97
Aubergine pizzas 206
Cauliflower rice 196
Chorizo and cauliflower soup 137
Eurodiet egg fried rice 150
Jambalaya 172
Lamb and feta burgers 168
Mushroom risotto with konjac
rice 198
Pilau cauliflower rice 201
Prawns with konjac spaghetti 171
Stir-fry with turmeric and chilli
215
Yuk sung with spicy cabbage
159–61
Stevia 70, 72
Stir-fry with turmeric and chilli 215
Strawberry and vanilla trifle 226
Stuffed courgettes 216
Stuffed tomatoes 156
sugar
alternatives to 72
fructose 130
fruit juices and 10
'hidden sugars' 69
insulin production and 41
milk sugar (lactose) 72, 98
sweet potatoes
Beef and red wine casserole 187
Cape Malay-style fish curry 186
Moussaka 181
Sweet potato and celeriac soup
144

**T**

Taylor, Roy 4
TOFI (thin outside, fat inside) 11,
12, 35, 39
Tofu 80
Tomato and bean soup 139
tomato passata
Chicken and aubergine bake 176
Spicy chicken and vegetable
casserole 158
Stuffed courgettes 216
tomato purée
Chicken and aubergine bake 176
Tomato and vegetable sauce 209
Vegetarian lasagne 190
Yellow peppers stuffed with feta
and pine nuts 191
tomatoes 60, 97
Beef and red wine casserole 187
Cape Malay-style fish curry 186

Chicken Caesar lettuce wrap 147
Chorizo and cauliflower soup 137
Italian-style roasted balsamic
    vegetables 208
Jambalaya 172
Moroccan spiced vegetables
    210–11
Moussaka 181
Pasta Bolognese 164
Stuffed tomatoes 156
Tomato and bean soup 139
Tomato and vegetable sauce
    209
Turkey and horseradish burgers
    175
Vegetarian lasagne 190
Yellow peppers stuffed with feta
    and pine nuts 191
tomatoes (sun-dried), Green lentil
    and pomegranate molasses salad
    126–8
Tropical breakfast smoothie 114
Turkey and horseradish burgers 175
turnips 60, 97
    Chicken and turnip curry 167
    Turnip chips with Cajun
        seasoning 202

**V**

Vegetable gratin 197
vegetables 60, 70, 72, 96, 97
Vegetarian burgers with tzatziki and
    quinoa 182–3
Vegetarian lasagne 190
venison sausages, Hunter's casserole
    188
Very Low Calorie Ketogenic Diet
    (VLCKD) 5, 53, 61–7
    alcohol and 48, 69
    BMI and 62
    caffeinated drinks 69
    calorie intake 63, 69
    carbohydrates 62, 67, 69
    chronic stress and 69–70
    constipation and 70–1
    Eurodiet products and 63–4, 72
    exercise and 69
    fats 62, 63
    glucose-lowering medication
        and 66, 67
    'hidden sugars' 69
    high-protein/low-carb diet 65
    insulin and 65–6
    ketone bodies and 63
    macronutrients 62–3
    medical issues 69

medical supervision and 62, 67
medication and 65–6, 69
menstrual cycle 69
micronutrients 63
plan, four phases to 72
protein 62, 64, 65
sleep and 69
slow weight loss, reasons for
    69–70
supplements and 63–4
weight loss and 68–9
vitamin K 60
vitamins 63, 64
VLCKD diet plan
    breakfast 74
    carbohydrates and 72
    cheeses and 98, 99
    dinner 75
    drinks and 72
    Eurodiet products 72, 73
    Laktolight 77
    lunch 74
    Maintenance Phase 72, 87–93
    Maintenance sample meal
        plan 93
    Phase (1) 72, 74–7, 97
    Phase (1) sample meal plan 76
    Phase (2) 72, 78–81, 97
    Phase (2) protein portion size 80
    Phase (2) sample meal plan 81
    Phase (3) 72, 82–5
    Phase (3) carbohydrates 84
    Phase (3) protein portion size 80
    Phase (3) sample meal plan 83
    snack times 74
    vegetables and 97

**W**

walnuts, Green lentil and
    pomegranate molasses salad 126–8
Warfarin (Coumadin) 60
Warm chicken and coconut salad 130
weight loss 7
    activity levels and 90–1
    benefits of 62
    BMI vs waist measurement
        38–40
    BMR and 89
    carbohydrates and 91–2
    maintenance and 87–92
    sleep and 69, 91
    slow weight loss 61, 68–9
    waist measurement 36, 38–40,
        46

wholemeal spelt flour, Fiery pizza
    with spicy pepperoni and jalapeño
    peppers 178–9
wholemeal wraps
        Buffalo chicken wrap pizza 131
        Chicken fajitas 192
wine, Beef and red wine casserole 187
Worcester sauce 156, 158, 177, 198

**X**

Xylitol 70, 72, 108, 146, 209, 211

**Y**

Yellow peppers stuffed with feta and
    pine nuts 191
Yellow vegetable curry with curly
    kale 214
yoghurt
        Chicken fajitas 192
        Lemon and raspberry
            cheesecakes 224
        Vegetarian burgers with tzatziki
            and quinoa 182–3
Yuk sung with spicy cabbage 159–61